Main

WHY YOU SHOULD READ THIS BOOK

Like most of us today, you probably have to carve out time in your busy schedule in order to find time to read a book. Therefore, you don't want your time to be wasted, and you want what you read to have value for you. Most likely, you are also looking for answers for how you can improve your health and the health of your loved ones. This is precisely why I wrote this book.

The plain truth is we are in the midst of a healthcare crisis. As a nation, we pay more per person for the medical care we receive, yet still have been unable to stem the rising tide of chronic degenerative diseases that afflict an ever growing percentage of our society. In addition, far too many of us rely on mainstream medicine to take care of our ills, without taking responsibility for maintaining our own health. Yet, there is much that we can do on our own to get and stay well, including learning about and using natural, inexpensive and proven treatments that can be as effective as any prescription or over-the-counter drug. One such effective treatment is the use of apple cider vinegar.

While the use of apple cider vinegar as an aid to improving and maintaining health may be unfamiliar to you, its use as a healing remedy for literally dozens of common health complaints has been documented all around the world for hundreds of years. In the pages that follow, you will learn just how effective apple cider vinegar can be for preventing and reversing over 80 health conditions, at least some of which most likely affect you or someone in your family.

If you read this book to its end and, most importantly, if you apply the suggestions for improving your health that it offers on a consistent basis, I promise you that your time will not be wasted and that there is a very good chance that you will find beneficial answers to your health concerns that will make a positive difference in your life.

Thank you for choosing to read it.

OTHER WORKS BY LARRY TRIVIERI, JR.

From Square One Publishers

*The Acid-Alkaline Lifestyle: The Complete Program
for Better Health and Vitality* (with Neil Raff, MD)

The Acid-Alkaline Food Guide
(with Susan Brown, PhD)

Juice Alive: The Ultimate Guide to Juicing Remedies
(with Steven Bailey, ND)

Other Select Titles

Alternative Medicine: The Definitive Guide, 1st and 2nd editions
(editor and co-author with Burton Goldberg)

The American Holistic Medical Association Guide to Holistic Health

Chronic Fatigue, Fibromyalgia and Lyme Disease
(with Burton Goldberg)

Novels

The Monster and Freddie Fype

Krystle's Quest

Tommy's Big Question

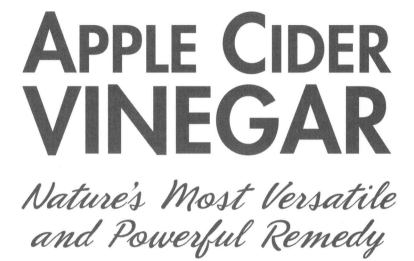

APPLE CIDER VINEGAR

Nature's Most Versatile and Powerful Remedy

Larry Trivieri, Jr.

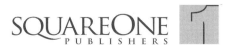

SQUAREONE
PUBLISHERS

The information and advice contained in this book are based upon the research and the personal and professional experiences of the authors. They are not intended as a substitute for consulting with a health care professional. The publisher and author are not responsible for any adverse effects or consequences resulting from the use of any of the suggestions, preparations, or procedures discussed in this book. All matters pertaining to your physical health should be supervised by a health care professional. It is a sign of wisdom, not cowardice, to seek a second or third opinion.

EDITOR: Erica Shur
COVER DESIGNER: Jeannie Tudor
TYPESETTER: Gary A. Rosenberg

Square One Publishers
115 Herricks Road
Garden City Park, NY 11040
(516) 535-2010 • (877) 900-BOOK
www.squareonepublishers.com

Library of Congress Cataloging-in-Publication Data
Names: Trivieri, Larry, 1956- author.
Title: Apple cider vinegar : nature's most versatile and powerful remedy / Larry Trivieri Jr.
Description: Garden City Park, NY : Square One Publishers, [2017] | Includes bibliographical references and index.
Identifiers: LCCN 2017013961 | ISBN 9780757004469
Subjects: LCSH: Cider vinegar—Therapeutic use—Popular works. | Cider vinegar—Health aspects—Popular works.
Classification: LCC RM666.V55 T75 2017 | DDC 615.3/23642—dc23
LC record available at https://lccn.loc.gov/2017013961
Copyright © 2017 by Larry Trivieri, Jr

Printed in the United States of America

10   9   8   7   6   5   4   3   2   1

Contents

For my niece,
Sonya Piersma,
who has a heart of gold.

Preface

For nearly 30 years I have devoted myself to researching and writing about the most effective and viable therapies and other healing approaches for reversing disease and creating and maintaining optimal health. My interest in health and healing began in the 1980s when, on two separate occasions, so-called alternative therapies quickly and completely healed me of two chronic conditions after months of conventional medical treatments had done nothing more than mitigate my symptoms. In the first instance, a single treatment by a very gifted acupuncturist cured me of chronic, debilitating bronchitis that had proven resistant to the drugs my family doctor had prescribed. In the second, a homeopathic remedy enabled me to easily and painlessly pass a lingering and sizeable kidney stone.

Because of those two experiences, I became intensely curious about such non-mainstream healthcare approaches and wondered why more people, especially physicians, did not utilize them. As a result, I spent the next few years reading about such therapies and seeking out practitioners who were skilled in them so that I could find out for myself whether or not they worked. Based on my experiences, I soon realized that these therapies did indeed work. Moreover, they did so without the side effects common to pharmaceutical drugs, and were also typically less expensive than most conventional medical approaches. From that point on in my life, I resolved to do whatever I could to tell as many people as possible about the discoveries I was making so that they would know the full range of healing options—both conventional *and* alternative—that were available to them.

Soon after I made that resolution, I met Burton Goldberg, the man who was destined to become not only my good friend, but also my most important mentor. Burton hired me to edit and co-author both the first and second editions of *Alternative Medicine: The Definitive Guide*, a landmark encyclopedic reference that covers more than 50 alternative medicine therapies and details how and why they could effectively treat more than 200 major health conditions, including AIDS, cancer, and heart disease. During the Guide's creation, I was privileged to meet and learn from approximately 400 of the most knowledgeable doctors and healers in the alternative medicine field. I also met and interviewed hundreds of their patients who shared with me their triumphs over a wide range of debilitating diseases after using such therapies. Many of their stories are included as inspiring case histories in the Guide. Within a year of its initial publication in 1994, the Guide, which Burton financed and self-published, became a major bestseller and today, more than 20 years later and with close to a million copies sold, it continues to help those seeking the most effective solutions to their health problems.

Following the publication of the Guide's first edition, I began to write my own books, including the only book ever to receive the official imprimatur of the American Holistic Medical Association (now the Academy of Integrative Health and Medicine), the nation's oldest organization advocating the use of alternative and integrative medicine, which was founded by the renowned Dr. C. Norman Shealy. My focus for the first books I wrote remained largely on professional care therapies within the alternative-integrative medicine umbrella. Over time, however, I came to realize that, despite how effective such therapies are, and even though there are a wide range of medical studies that have proven their effectiveness, by and large most of them remain largely unknown to the average American and, more importantly, are not available to them due to the fact that in many areas of the United States such practitioners are not to be found. (Notable exceptions include chiropractors, clinical nutritionists—which are different than dieticians—body workers, massage therapists, yoga and meditation instructors, and, perhaps, herbalists and acupuncturists.) And even if such practitioners are available in your area, for the most part—again with certain exceptions—the therapies and other services they provide are not covered by health insurance (primarily due to the stranglehold the pharmaceutical industry, sadly with the collusion of both federal and state government agencies, have on our nation's symptom-management "healthcare" system.)

Recognizing these facts, over time, my focus as a writer has increasingly shifted to writing about effective self-care, rather than professional care, approaches and remedies that are widely available to everyone, which can be used both to prevent and reverse disease, and which, just as importantly, will not make a dent in your wallet or pocketbook. So it was that I have teamed up with various doctors and other health experts to co-author or ghostwrite books on such topics as juicing, probiotics, various nutritional supplements, and diet, specifically with a focus on eating in a way that supports optimal acid-alkaline (pH) balance in the body. All told, I've written nearly 20 books on such subjects, and continue to keep an eye out for other effective self-care methods that my readers can benefit from.

Yet, until recently, I completely overlooked one of the oldest, least expensive, and most versatile healing remedies—apple cider vinegar. This book makes amends for that.

I had heard of the healing properties of apple cider vinegar for years, and I've long used it on the salads I make and eat on a regular basis. Dr. Susan Brown and I also included it in our bestselling book, *The Acid-Alkaline Food Guide* because of its proven alkalizing benefits. Beyond that, though, I hadn't paid much attention to whatever other possible benefits it was claimed to have.

That all changed when someone I know cured himself of a long-standing case of GERD (gastro-esophageal reflux disease) simply by drinking a few glasses of water each day, to which he'd added a few capfuls of apple cider vinegar. What was most remarkable about the resolution of his condition was that everything else he had tried, including significant changes in his diet, had offered him no relief whatsoever, leaving him to suffer from his condition for months.

Although many doctors and researchers might dismiss this case as being merely anecdotal, I long ago learned to pay attention to such anecdotes because oftentimes they can offer clues to solutions that modern science has not taken an interest in. Intrigued by this person's turnaround, I decided that maybe I should take a closer look into what potential benefits apple cider could provide. As I did so, I discovered its use as a healing agent dates back thousands of years. Even more surprising to me was my discovery that there actually *are* a number of scientific studies attesting to apple cider vinegar's health-promoting properties in relation to various health conditions. In short, I realized apple cider's numerous benefits deserved to be known by as many people as possible. This book is my effort to help make that happen. I hope that it will empower you to take better control over your health and the health of your loved ones.

Introduction

Imagine a drug that came to market after being shown that it could safely and effectively:

- Boost your immune function and improve your resistance to infectious disease
- Help prevent and treat high blood pressure
- Help prevent and reverse high cholesterol
- Reduce the risk of diabetes
- Help regulate blood sugar levels
- Reduce inflammation
- Relieve allergies
- Soothe away arthritis and joint pains
- Alleviate muscle cramps
- Help prevent bone loss
- Help prevent and treat colds and flu
- Reduce the risk of cataracts
- Improve your digestion and overall gastrointestinal function
- Improve bladder, kidney, and liver function
- Increase your energy levels and reduce fatigue
- Boost your metabolism and aid in weight loss

And that's just the tip of the apple. It can also help prevent and treat scores of other common health conditions, ranging from back pain, congestion, constipation, and diarrhea to headache, heartburn, urinary tract infections, varicose veins, and yeast infections, plus, in the process, also improve the appearance of your skin and improve the luster and sheen of your hair, all without any side effects whatsoever.

If such a drug existed, surely millions of patients would flock to their doctors demanding that they be given a prescription for it. Most likely, you would be one of them. And because of the multitude of benefits the drug provided, the drug company that brought it to market could expect to reap annual profits of hundreds of millions, and perhaps even billions, of dollars.

But such a drug does not exist, nor is there ever likely to be one, for the simple reason that pharmaceutical drugs are designed to only target specific and limited mechanisms in the body, thereby significantly narrowing the scope of what such drugs can treat. Moreover, few, if any drugs, have much value as a preventive agent, and all of them, even common aspirin, pose the risk of harmful side effects.

Fortunately, however, you don't have to wish that someday a scientist might discover a drug that *did* provide all of the benefits listed above. Instead, you can turn to Mother Nature, for she has already provided us with a substance that can do all of the above and much more. That substance is apple cider vinegar. (Hereinafter, I will sometimes refer to apple cider vinegar by its abbreviation, ACV.)

It's likely, however, that until now you have not been aware of just how powerful and versatile apple cider vinegar is as a healing agent for so many health conditions. The reason for this is simple.

Unlike pharmaceutical drugs, which, in the United States, are heavily marketed to the public via a bombardment of ads on television, radio, newspapers, magazines, and the Internet (only the U.S. and New Zealand allow this type of direct-to-consumer drug advertising, by the way), in addition to being the primary recommendation of most conventionally trained physicians to their patients, producers of apple cider vinegar are actually prevented by law from making any health claims about ACV. If they did so, they would soon face heavy fines by federal agencies such as the Food and Drug Administration (FDA) and the Federal Trade Commission (FTC), and might even be forced out of business. (In fact, our nation's laws with regard to health claims are so draconian that the FDA literally controls the definition of the word "drug," meaning that anytime a health claim is made about a natural healing substance, the FDA can and does assert that said substance is being marketed as a drug, and therefore subject to the same fines and other legal penalties that drug companies face when they make what the FDA terms "unsubstantiated claims." These same hurdles and restrictions are also imposed on most producers of nutritional supplements and other natural products.)

Moreover, ACV producers, even if they were allowed to do so, have no incentive to finance the types of studies that pharmaceutical companies underwrite to bring their drugs to market (the cost of doing so today is estimated to be as high as $800 million or more for a single drug before it can secure FDA approval) because, unlike such drugs, ACV cannot be patented. (Patented drugs, once approved by the FDA, enable the pharmaceutical companies that develop them to reap billions of dollars in annual profits by exclusively selling the drugs under brand names for a period of up to 20 years. Only after this exclusivity period expires are competing drugs companies allowed to bring generic versions of these drugs to market. This is one of the reasons why pharmaceutical drugs are so expensive—because they have the exclusive right to sell their drugs for so many years, drug companies typically are allowed to charge whatever to want for the drugs during that exclusivity period—and also a primary reason why are nation's annual healthcare costs today total $3 trillion, a figure that continues to increase.)

For these and other reasons, it's unlikely that you will find much, if any, advertising about apple cider vinegar. Instead, the companies which produce and sell it are content to simply place their bottles of ACV in the condiment aisles of grocery and health food stores across the country, where they continue to sell because, after all, nearly everyone uses ACV from time to time as an ingredient for salad dressing. Savvy, health conscious individuals, however, also regularly stock up on ACV because they know of at least some of the other health-promoting benefits that ACV provides and which you will discover by reading this book.

In the pages that follow, you will learn about apple cider vinegar's long history as a healing agent. You will then discover how and why it works, including what modern science has discovered about its healing properties, along with guidelines for knowing what to look for when choosing an apple cider vinegar product. You will also learn how, if you are so inclined, you can make your own supply of apple cider vinegar at home. Most importantly, you will discover how to use apple cider vinegar to treat more than 80 common health conditions, along with its various other uses.

Of course, no single ingredient, even one as powerful and versatile as apple cider vinegar has proven to be, can serve as a "magic bullet" when it comes to your health. For this reason, this book also includes a variety of other important and easy-to-implement self-care approaches you can apply as part of your daily health routine.

Now that you know that apple cider vinegar can act as a multipurpose health aid, let's take a look at what ACV actually is, how and why it works, and the many ways that it can improve your health.

PART ONE

Apple Cider Vinegar— The Ancient Healer

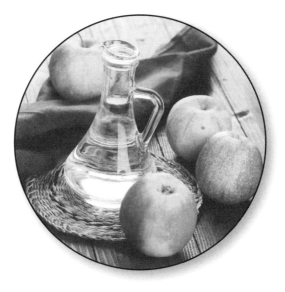

1.

Apple Cider Vinegar— The Versatile Healer

Apple cider vinegar is one variety of vinegar itself, a substance that has been in use for thousands of years. The word *vinegar* is derived from the French words *vin aigre*, which translate as "sour wine." Vinegar was so named because many of types of vinegar are produced from diluted wines, as well as other diluted forms of alcohol. Long before the French gave it its current name, however, vinegar was used for a variety of purposes all throughout the world.

Essentially, anything that can be fermented is capable of producing vinegar, which is why today there are many varieties of vinegar, ranging from common white vinegar (distilled from grains) and apple cider vinegar, to red and white wine vinegars, rice vinegar, and balsamic vinegar, to sherry, malt, and champagne vinegars. There are even vinegars derived from dates (quite possibly the earliest form of vinegar in history), sugar cane, raisins, coconuts, pomegranates, and honey.

WHAT IS APPLE CIDER VINEGAR?

Apple cider vinegar (ACV), of course, as its name implies, is derived from apples. It is produced by a two-stage fermentation process. In the first stage, apples are added to water and combined with yeast or sugar. The apples ferment together with the yeast or sugar to produce alcohol. Once this occurs, the second stage begins during which bacteria is added to change the alcohol into vinegar. The vinegar is then allowed to mature, becoming a rich brown in color and containing a foamy, bacteria-laden substance known as the "mother," an ingredient that is responsible for many of ACV's health benefits and which is found in the best ACV products. (You will learn more about the "mother" and why it is so important in Chapter 2, and in Chapter 4 you will learn how you can easily produce your own apple cider vinegar at home.)

During this fermentation process, a substance known as acetic acid, also known as glacial acetic acid, is produced. Acetic acid is found in all forms of vinegar, typically in concentrations of 3 to 9 percent by volume. Apart from water, acetic acid is the main component of apple cider vinegar, and is a primary reason why ACV is so healthy for you. Various other bioactive compounds are also found in apple cider vinegar, all of which you will learn more about in Chapter 2.

VINEGAR THROUGH THE AGES

Let's turn our attention to the uses of vinegar, including apple cider vinegar, throughout history. You may be surprised, as I was, to discover that the use of vinegars, including ACV, for healing dates back thousands of years.

Early Origins

The earliest known use of vinegar can be traced back to the Mesopotamian civilizations of early recorded history, beginning with the Ubaid and Uruks, and then followed, successively, by the empires of Sumer, Assyria, Akkadia, and Babylon. Legend has it that a courtier around 5, 000 BCE accidentally discovered wine after coming upon a batch of grape juice that had been unattended and thus had fermented. The discovery of vinegar from wine soon followed. Whether the anecdote of the courier is true or not, records from that time period reveal that the peoples from that time were producing vinegar from date palm fruits, honey, and malt, and using it in their food, as well as a preservative and a pickling agent, and that the Babylonians were producing and selling various types of vinegar from the 18th to 6th century BCE.

The use of vinegar soon spread to neighboring Egypt and other regions in the Middle East. Residues of vinegar, for example, have been found in Egyptian urns dating as far back as 3, 000 BCE. References to the health benefits of vinegar can also be found in the writings preserved from ancient Middle Eastern cultures. In them vinegar is mentioned as a medicinal aid for a variety of conditions, including digestion problems, respiratory conditions, and for dressing wounds and preventing them from becoming infected. It was also commonly used as a condiment.

Vinegar In The Bible

Vinegar is also mentioned numerous times in both the Old and New Testaments of the Christian Bible. For example, in the Book of Ruth (2:14), Ruth, after toiling all day in the fields during harvest season, is invited by the wealthy landowner Boaz to have dinner, saying "Come here, that you may eat of the bread and dip your piece of bread in the vinegar." This is an example of how, during biblical times, vinegar was used by the Jewish people as a condiment that added flavor to food. In the New Testament, perhaps the most well-known mention of vinegar occurs during the crucifixion of Jesus. In the

Gospel of John (19:28-30), it is written, "Later, knowing that everything had now been finished, and so that Scripture would be fulfilled, Jesus said, 'I am thirsty.' A jar of wine vinegar was there, so they soaked a sponge in it, put the sponge on a stalk of the hyssop plant, and lifted it to Jesus' lips." Though this offering of vinegar is often construed to mean that Jesus was being mocked, in actuality, at that time, this mixture of vinegar was commonly used by Roman soldiers and workers as an energizing tonic known as *posca*.

Ancient Greece and Rome

From the Middle East, the use of vinegar spread to both the ancient Greek and Roman civilizations. Records show, for instance, that by 1, 000 BCE vinegar was commonly being produced in ancient Rome from wine, dates, figs, and other fruits, and used as an additive to drinking water. Vinegar bowls was also commonly used during meals so that bread could be dipped into them. Meanwhile, in Greece, approximately 2,500 years ago, Hippocrates, the Father of Western Medicine, also advocated the use of vinegar for healing. It is in the writings of Hippocrates that we find some of the earliest recommendations for the use of apple cider vinegar for healing. He prescribed it for a variety of conditions, including coughs and colds. Hippocrates also recommended vinegar as an antiseptic aid for cleaning and treating wounds. He was also one of the first Western healers to combine ACV with honey to be consumed as an overall health tonic.

During the time of the Roman Empire, military generals, including Julius Caesar, had their troops consume vinegar diluted in water (posca) for its energizing tonic properties. Vinegar was also carried by the Roman armies in their military campaigns because of its effectiveness as a disinfectant when added to drinking water from foreign lands. This was documented in Julius Caesar's *Commentarii de Bello Gallico* (Commentaries on the Gallic War), his firsthand account of his nine-year campaign against the Germanic and Celtic armies in Gaul (modern-day northern Italy, France, Belgium, Luxemburg, western Germany, and most of Switzerland), which he wrote between the years 58 and 50 BCE. Another piece of Roman literature, the extensive cookbook *De Re Coquinaria* (On the Subject of Cooking), which dates back to about the year 230 CE, includes the use of vinegar in approximately 150 recipes, indicating that the use of vinegar was quite common and popular in everyday Roman kitchens.

Ancient Asia

Centuries before the dawn of the Roman Empire, vinegar was already in use in Asia. The earliest references to vinegar use in China occurred during the

Two Curious Tales About Vinegar

Two of the most curious uses of vinegar come to us from the ancient Roman historians Titus Livius (also known as Livy) and Pliny the Elder (Gaius Plinius Secundus). The first is recounted by Livy in his *Ab Urbe Conditi Libri* (Books from the Foundation of the City), a series of works documenting the history of ancient Rome. Included in the works is an account of how the famed Hannibal of Carthage used vinegar to find a way through a cliff of boulders that blocked the advance of his army. Livy writes, "The soldiers were then forced to find a passage through the cliff, which was the only traversable way, and because the rocks should be broken, they felled and cut many large trees growing around, erected a huge pile of timber and set fire to it with the favor of a strong wind that excited the flames and, pouring vinegar on the heated stones, they broke them into small crumbs."

In his work *Naturalis Historia* (Natural History), which became the model for subsequent encyclopedias, Pliny the Elder describes how the Egyptian queen, Cleopatra, showed off her wealth during a banquet held for the Roman general Marc Antony (Marcus Antonius), who was destined to become her lover. During the banquet, Cleopatra wagered with Antony that she could consume a fortune during the course of the meal. Once the wager was accepted, Pliny writes, "According to given orders, the servants set before her a vase of vinegar, the sharpness and strength of which is able to dissolve pearls. She was wearing in her ears those choicest and most rare and unique productions of nature. Then, while Antony was waiting to see what she was going to do, she took one of them off, dipped it into vinegar and, once dissolved, she swallowed it." And so she won her bet.

Zhou Dynasty (1027–221 BCE). The most famous ancient account of that period of China's history is the *Zhu Zhuan* (also sometimes spelled *Tso Chuan*), which mentions a flavoring and condiment called *liu*, which historians have interpreted to mean vinegar.

The medicinal properties of vinegar were recognized around the same time, including by Song Ci (1186–1249 CE), one of the most noteworthy persons in China's early history. Song Ci, a Confucian scholar, is known as "the father of forensic medicine." He served many terms as a presiding judge in the Chinese high courts, and made a point of personally examining crime scenes each time he encountered a difficult case of homicide or physical assault. As a result of his investigations, he combined many historical cases of forensic science with his own experiences to write the book *Xi Yuan Ji Lu* (Collected Cases of Injustice Rectified) in the hopes that it would help other judges avoid miscarriages of justice. This book continues to be highly regarded by forensic scientists today.

Song Ci's connection to vinegar rests on the fact that, more than six hundred years before the Hungarian physician Ignaz Semmelweis introduced the practice of hand washing to Western doctors before and after treating their patients in order prevent infection, Song Ci advocated the same practice so as to prevent infection during autopsies. In order to do so, he advised that hands be washed with a mixture of vinegar and sulfur. (Semmelweis recommended using a chlorinated lime solution.)

It is interesting to note that Song Ci's recommendation was readily accepted by the Chinese, whereas Semmelweis was ridiculed and harassed by his medical colleagues, and dismissed from the hospital in which he worked. Outraged by the rejection of his commonsense recommendation by the medical profession, he began writing open and increasingly angry letters to prominent European physicians, going so far to denounce them as irresponsible murderers. His growing sense of anger led many, including his wife, to believe he was losing his mind and he was eventually committed to an asylum, where he died only 14 days later. It was only after Louis Pasteur developed the germ theory of disease years later that Semmelweis' recommendation was finally widely adopted by Western doctors. Today, Semmelweis is considered a pioneer of antiseptic procedures, while, in the West, historians overlook the fact that, Song Ci introduced them centuries earlier.

By the 14th century, during the Ming Dynasty, vinegar was recognized and used as both an internal and external cleansing agent. In 1368, the Chinese medical treatise *Yin shih Hsu chih* (Essential Knowledge of Eating and Cooking) emphasized the importance of disease prevention, and recommended the use of vinegar to counteract the effects of tainted fish, meat, fruit, and vegetables. By 1381, the increased demand for vinegar throughout China caused the government to establish a bureau solely dedicated to overseeing the production and distribution of vinegar.

In classical Chinese cooking, which has its roots in ancient China, vinegar was, and continues to be, used as a primary ingredient to prepare a wide variety of Chinese dishes, which are known for their "five flavors" (sweet, sour, salty, pungent, and bitter). Vinegar is primarily used in dishes in the sour and bitter categories.

Diet is an essential component of traditional Chinese medicine (TCM), one of the world's oldest and most comprehensive systems of medicine. TCM practitioners make little distinction between food and medicine, recognizing that both are derived from the same original sources. In that regard, they very much adhere to Hippocrates' famous dictum, "Let food be thy medicine, and medicine thy food."

According to TCM theory, vinegar has numerous medicinal benefits. Bob Flaws, Dipl. Ac. & C.H., FNAAOM, author of *The Tao of Healthy Eating: Dietary Wisdom According to Chinese Medicine,* explains that vinegar "enters the liver and stomach channels, and its functions are that it scatters stasis, stops bleeding, resolves toxins, and kills worms. In professional Chinese medicine, various Chinese medicinals are stir-fried in vinegar in order to either help target them to the liver-gallbladder or to increase their functions of moving the Qi [vital life force energy; pronounced "chee"] and quickening the blood. However, in Chinese folk medicine, vinegar is a medicinal in its own right, treating a wide range of disorders and complaints, including internal medicine, gynecological, dermatological, and traumatological conditions."

Since ancient times, both practitioners of TCM, as well as Chinese folk healers, have used vinegar to help treat literally hundreds of disease conditions, including indigestion and other digestive problems, dysentery, hepatitis, arteriosclerosis and coronary heart disease, angina, diabetes, headache, edema, obesity, insomnia, and gingivitis, among many other health problems.

Vinegar's reputation as a healing agent in China grew during the 17th century because of a Buddhist monk in Sichuan, who lived to be over 100 years old. His longevity was said to be due to a vinegar-based herbal drink that he consumed daily throughout his long life. It was believed that this beverage cured his colds and protected him from infectious disease.

The most popular form of vinegar in ancient China, which is still very popular today, was rice vinegar, which was used as a flavoring well before the advent of the Christian era. Rice vinegar is also very popular in Japan, and historians have established that rice vinegar methods that originated in China traveled to Japan as early as 270 CE. Known as *komesu* in Japan, rice vinegar was taxed as a form of sake as early as the 8th century CE. By the 1600s, rice vinegar was widely in use throughout Japan, and continues to be so today.

Finally, it is also worth noting that during the era of the Japanese Samurai, which lasted for approximately 700 years (1185 to 1868), Samurai regularly consumed rice vinegar mixed with water to boost their strength, much like the soldiers of the earlier Roman legions drank *posca* for the same purpose.

Islamic World

Just as it was in other cultures around the world by this time, vinegar was widely used in Muslim countries. Islam, which was founded on the teachings of the Prophet Muhammad in the 7th century, was notable for producing many scientific advances at a time when much of Europe remained steeped in ignorance and superstition. Additionally, even though the use of vinegar spread during the Middle Ages in Europe, because of the crucifixion scene in the New Testament in which Jesus was offered vinegar on a sponge, Christian writers of the time typically associated vinegar with fraud, deceit, and mental corruption. One example of this comes from the *De Rerum Naturis* (On the Natures of Things), written by Rabanus Maurus Magnentius, a 9th century German archbishop. In it, he writes, "In a mystical sense, vinegar itself represents the corrupted purity of mind, thus in the Psalm it is said, 'and in my thirst they gave me vinegar to drink'." Given that Rabanus was called "the teacher of Germany," his writings were greatly influential at the time.

By contrast, among Muslims vinegar was highly regarded because of how favorably it is mentioned in sacred Islamic texts, such as the *Kitab Al-Ashriba* (The Book of Drinks), in which Muhammad is quoted as saying, "Vinegar is a good condiment." Vinegar, as well, has always been considered *halal* (allowed) by Muslims, even when it is produced from wine, which is strictly forbidden by their religion.

Overall, Islamic scientists and scholars during this period had a superior knowledge and understanding of chemistry and other sciences than their European counterparts. Two of the most noteworthy Islamic scientists of the time were Abu Musa Jabir Ibn Hayyan (721–815), known in the West by his Latin name, Geber, and the famed scientist and healer Ibn Sina (980–1037), who is better known today as Avicenna.

Geber is considered the "Father of Chemistry" for the advances he made in that science. In addition to his skills as a chemist, he was also an astronomer, engineer, geographer, physicist, pharmacist, and a physician and wrote numerous texts during his lifetime, a number of which were translated into Latin and became standard reference texts for European scientists. Among his many contributions to science was his extensive study of vinegar and its properties. Geber was also the discoverer of acetic acid. His discovery came about when he distilled acetic acid out of vinegar. Today, we know that acetic acid, one of vinegar's main components, is responsible for its many healing properties.

Like Geber, Avicenna was highly accomplished in a variety of disciplines, including astronomy, geography, geology, logic, mathematics, medicine, physics, psychology, and theology. He was also an accomplished poet, and is regarded as one of the most important figures of the Golden Age of Islam.

During his lifetime, Avicenna wrote 450 works, including 40 texts on medicine. Of these, his most famous and influential works are *Kitab Al-Shifa* (The Book of Healing) and the five volume encyclopedia *Al-Qanun fi't-Tibb*

(The Canon of Medicine), which was translated into Latin and was a standard medical reference text in universities throughout medieval Europe right up through the mid-17th century. And it is still regarded as an essential reference today by practitioners of Unani medicine, a traditional system of healing practiced in Muslim cultures in India and other Asian countries. Avicenna wrote about vinegar's healing properties in both of these works, recommending it as a digestive aid, an expectorant, a highly effective clotting agent, and a balm for skin inflammations and burns. He also found it effective for relieving headaches caused by heat when applied topically.

In Medieval Europe

The medieval period of European history spans a thousand years, beginning in the 5th century, following the decline of the Roman Empire and the dawn of the Middle ages, and culminating in the 15th century with the Renaissance, also known as the Age of Discovery. By its end, there had been an explosion of shared knowledge throughout Europe, in large part due to the invention of Gutenberg's printing press and the widespread dissemination of books and other written documents. Additionally, beginning in the 14th century, many of the written works of medicine, as well as many other disciplines, that originated in the Islamic world were translated into Latin, adding to the stores of knowledge in the West.

It was during this period of medieval history that further advances in the production of vinegar occurred. One of the most noteworthy was the invention of balsamic vinegar in Italy. The first historical reference to balsamic vinegar dates back to 1046 in a document that records that a bottle of balsamic vinegar was given as a gift to Emperor Enrico III of Franconia (modern day Bavaria in Germany.) Following its invention, balsamic vinegar became a popular condiment, and throughout the Middle Ages it was also used as a disinfectant. Many healers of the time also ascribed many other medicinal uses for it, ranging from colds and sore throats to labor pains.

As vinegar grew in popularity throughout all of Western Europe because of its many uses, the demand for it crippled its supply, because at the time it was largely homemade and was not being produced in large quantities. Thus it was only obtainable on a small scale. Yet the demand for it did not diminish.

The problem of supply was solved in 1394, thanks to a group of French wine merchants from Orleans, France, who developed a new way of producing vinegar. It became known as the Orleans method, and enabled vinegar to be produced continuously, rather than by the previous method of producing it in one small batch at a time. The Orleans method, sometimes referred to as the "continuous method," is still in use today. It originally involved slowly fermenting wine in wooden barrels or casks to produce vinegar. Once the vinegar was produced, it was siphoned off through a spigot at the bottom of each cask, with approximately 15 percent of the vinegar left behind. The remaining vinegar contained the "mother vinegar," with its concentrated bacteria floating on top. Small amounts of this "mother vinegar" was then added to new barrels of wine to quick start the production of batches of vinegar. Then, as the new vinegar it produced reached its desired flavor and acidity, it was removed from the top of the barrels, to be replaced by fresh batches of wine so that the process could continuously repeat itself. Because of this method, the process of fermentation never stopped, allowing each production facility to always have new supplies of vinegar on hand.

This new production method was considered so valuable that the French government awarded the Orleans merchants an official statute that enabled them to form a corporation that soon resulted in them having a near monopoly over vinegar production, because they kept their production method secret. This, in turn, resulted in the creation of the French saying, *C'est le secret du vinaigrier* (it's the secret of the vinegar maker). Eventually the Orleans merchants formed a guild of master vinegar makers and grew rich as they used their method to meet the demand for their vinegar products.

The invention of the Orleans method eventually led to the rise of a flourishing vinegar industry throughout Europe, which introduced scores of vinegar products, including many vinegars infused with spices, herbs, and fruits. By the 1700s, Europeans could choose from more than one hundred varieties of infused vinegars. In that same century, English merchants adapted the Orleans method to produce malt vinegar by fermenting ale. (Malt ale, also known as *alegar*, was also produced during the Middle Ages in the same fashion that other vinegars were prior to the invention of the Orlean method.) This led to the formation, in 1641, of a large production facility in London, which became the world's first "vinegar yard."

The time of the Black Plague, which raged on and off throughout Europe from 1347 to 1771, also revealed the healing properties of vinegar. The plague was highly contagious and very often fatal. During that time, physicians and others who tended the sick would rub vinegar infused with herbs and oils on their bodies to protect themselves from becoming infected. They would also cover the inside of their clothes with the same solutions of vinegar to further protect themselves.

Further evidence of the belief in vinegar's healing properties during the plague can be found in Derby, England. At the time, it was thought that the exchange of money (in the form of coins) could also spread the infection. To protect against this, a stone trough was placed in the market place of Derby and filled with vinegar. Money for goods and any change were placed in the stone so that the vinegar could act as a disinfectant and so prevent the spread of the disease. Known as the "vinegar stone" or the "headless cross," the stone still stands in Friars Gate in Derby today.

Another account of the power of vinegar to protect against the plague can be found in the book *Vinegars of the World,* edited by Laura Solieri and Paulo Giudici. It states, "In 1791, when the plague was spreading in France, a chronicle recounts that the homes of the disease victims were being raided by thieves. Nobody attempted to find them because they were expected to die soon, but as time went on the robberies did not stop and it was clear that the thieves were able to avoid catching the plague by using some kind of trick. The thieves were later identified: they were four boys and, when they were captured, the authorities offered to spare their lives if they revealed their secret weapon against the plague, so they had no choice. They revealed that their mother used to prepare a disinfectant brew made of vinegar, garlic, lavender, rosemary, mint, and other herbs; after pouring it over their bodies or bathing in it, they were not infected by the killer disease. This concoction then became famous under the name of 'Four Thieves Vinegar' and is still manufactured today, mainly in France."

During the Industrial Age and Into the 20th Century

The end of the medieval period also saw the discovery of the Americas by the Europeans. As they settled in the "New World," the production and use of vinegar came with them. During the 1600s, American colonists began to make apple cider due to the plentiful supply of wild apples they found in their new home. Allowing the cider to ferment, they also brewed the alcoholic hard cider beverage. Further fermentation produced apple cider vinegar, which was used by the colonists as a condiment, a natural medicine, a pickling agent, a preservative of fresh vegetables, and as a drink very much like the Roman soldiers' *posca* (apple cider diluted in water). It was also commonly used for cleaning and various other household chores.

Meanwhile, in Europe, where the Orleans method remained the sole industrial means of vinegar production right up until the 19th centuries, researchers continued to investigate the chemical properties of vinegar and to explore exactly how it was produced. In 1807, the French chemist and statesman Jean-Antoine Chapel (1756–1832), became the first person to comprehensively explain how the Orleans method worked from a scientific perspective. Around the same time, the British physicist Humphrey Davy (1778–1829) proved that it was the transformation of alcohol into acetic acid that was responsible for the production of vinegar. Davy also discovered the chemical formula for acetic acid.

Additional discoveries from that time included that of the Dutch scientist Christian Persoon, who in 1822 identified the main agent of the acetification process, which he named *Mycoderma aceti*. As often happens, however, Persoon's discovery that this microorganism was responsible for making vinegar was initially rejected and continued to be for another 40 years, by scientists who insisted that the fermentation process was entirely inorganic and spontaneous. In 1862, however, Persoon was vindicated when Louis Pasteur (1822–1895), the inventor of the "germ theory of disease," confirmed Persoon's findings. Pasteur went on to add to our knowledge of vinegar by not only proving that fermentation is caused by the spread of *Mycoderma aceti* (later known as *Acetobacter aceti*) and other microorganisms, but that it also oxidized alcohol to become acetic acid, and that this certainly was not a spontaneous process. Moreover, Pasteur, working with cultures of yeast, discovered that, while air should be prevented from interacting with fermenting wine, air was absolutely required in order to produce vinegar. Based on his experiments, Pasteur theorized that the vinegar production process could be improved by adding a defined measure of *Acetobacter aceti* and other microorganisms during the fermentation process.

The discoveries by Pasteur, Persoon, and others led to further innovations in vinegar production, especially with the dawn of the 20th century, when significant advances occurred, both in terms of equipment and in culturing processes. With the advent of these advances, the production of vinegar became even more efficient and less expensive, resulting in it becoming even more widely available. This was fortunate, since during World War I, with antibiotic drugs still to be discovered, vinegar was needed in great quantities, as it was used as a primary treatment for cleaning soldiers' wound and preventing the spread of infection.

As this section illustrates, vinegar in its various forms has had a very long and fascinating history, and has served as a staple product in many cultures and countries around the world. Now let's turn our attention back to apple cider vinegar specifically, particularly as it has been used in America.

APPLE CIDER VINEGAR IN AMERICA

The story of apple cider vinegar in America in many ways begins with the pilgrims and other colonists from England who settled in the northeastern colonies in the 1600s. Although various varieties of wild crab apples were already native to North America at the time, it was these English settlers, who carried apple seeds with them during their journey to the New World, who introduced many of the apple varieties that we know and eat today.

The first colonist to do so was the English clergyman William Blackstone (also known as William Blaxton), who is claimed to have planted the first European strain of apple tree in the colonies. He planted it in Boston in 1623. In 1635, Blackstone moved to what is today known as Rhode Island, becoming its first European settler. In the same year, he planted an entire apple orchard in Rhode Island. He is also responsible for producing America's first native, non-crab apple variety, known as Blaxton's Yellow Sweeting.

Thanks to Blackstone and other settlers, the planting of apple trees continued to spread across much of the northern colonies. Before long, apples became a staple among the settlers, who not only ate them and fed them to their livestock, but also used them for cooking and other uses, including pressing them to make apple juice. In many cases, in turn, the apple juice was set aside and allowed to naturally ferment to become hard apple cider, a drink that was widely consumed by New Englanders at that time, including older children. So popular was apple cider in the region that by the time of the American Revolution a century later, it was estimated that 10 percent of all New England farms owned and operated their own cider mills. In fact, New Englander John Adams (1735–1826), one of the original signers of the Declaration of Independence and the second president of the United States, began each day with a drink of apple cider.

Not all batches of apple cider were consumed, however. Some were allowed to ferment even further, to produce apple cider vinegar, which also became widely used at the time, including as a form of natural medicine for a variety of health conditions ranging from colds and sore throats to arthritis, and as a disinfectant on wounds. ACV was also widely used as a condiment, pickling agent, and preservative, as well as for cleaning and other household chores.

Just as other types of vinegar had been used for centuries in Europe and elsewhere to treat the wounds of soldiers and prevent infection, so too was ACV use by some regiments of the American Revolutionary Army, a practice that continued both during the American Civil War by both the Union and Confederate armies, and into World War I. During these conflicts, American soldiers also consumed ACV with water or juice to prevent and relieve indigestion and other gastrointestinal problems, to protect against infectious disease, including pneumonia, and to prevent scurvy.

During the 1700s, apple cider vinegar became the primary ingredient of an energizing tonic drink consumed by many New England farmers during their daily labors. The tonic was known as *switchel*, also called "switzel" or "swizzle," and was made up of apple cider vinegar mixed with water or juice and sometimes with added honey. Ginger was sometimes also included as a seasoning. By the 1800s, switchel became a popular drink among farmers across many American states, especially during haying season. Because of how widely consumed it was by thirsty farmers as they harvested hay, switchel gained the nickname "haymaker's punch."

Following the American Revolution, the popularity of apple cider and apple cider vinegar continued to grow, and spread to other regions of the United States. By the early 1800s, thanks in large part to John Chapman (1774– 1845), better known to us as Johnny Appleseed, apple orchards and nurseries were growing as far west as Ohio, Indiana, Illinois, and in Virginia as well as up north in Ontario, Canada.

Chapman was a pioneer nurseryman and leading conservationist in America, beginning in his native Pennsylvania, where he was highly regarded because of his generous nature. He shared apple and other seeds with many frontier settlers, and planted many apple nurseries himself during his travels. Chapman was also a Christian missionary, who lived very simply and often traveled barefoot. To him, apples symbolized the bounty of God's creation, and as he traveled, he would often sing a hymn, which included the verse, "Oh, the Lord is good to me, and so I thank the Lord for giving me the things I need, the sun and the rain and the apple seed. The Lord is good to me. Amen." Because of his legacy, this verse is still said before mealtimes by some American families today.

By this time, because of how widely available both apple cider and apple cider vinegar had become in the United States, they both became popular units of exchange in place of money, especially in farming communities where currency was not always in use because of its scarcity in such rural areas. As a result, many farmers began producing far more apple cider and ACV than they needed, so that both could be used as payment for the goods and services they required, including livestock, other foodstuffs, and professional services. Even many rural doctors were paid this way. Of the two liquid "currencies," apple cider vinegar, on average, had a worth that was three times higher than apple cider.

Meanwhile, in the growing American cities of the 1800s, due to lack of indoor plumbing and modern sewage methods, the streets were ripe with the foul odors of raw sewage and other waste products. To counteract having to breathe this foul air and becoming sickened by it, the practice of soaking small sponges in apple cider vinegar soon arose. The sponges were held to the nose as people traveled through the city streets and carried in small silver boxes known as vinaigrettes. Many men stored their ACV-soaked sponges in small compartments in the heads of walking cans that were devised especially for this purpose.

Based on surviving medical texts dating from the late 18th and early 19th centuries, we know that medical practitioners across the United States commonly used apple cider vinegar as a primary treatment for numerous health conditions. These included stomach and gastrointestinal problems, croup, pneumonia and other respiratory conditions, colds and flu, fever, wounds, poison ivy, and dropsy (known today as edema). People who suffered from diabetes at the time also commonly drank teas to which ACV was added in order to help manage their diabetic symptoms.

In 1909, D.C. Jarvis, M.D., a Vermont physician, began to study the effectiveness of early American folk remedies, including apple cider vinegar. Based on his research, he soon began to regard ACV as a "cure-all" for nearly all health conditions. He advised his patients to take ACV as a digestive tonic with meals, writing that it aided digestion and destroyed harmful bacteria in the gastrointestinal tract. He also recommended combining ACV with honey in order to enhance its healing abilities, naming the mixture "honegar."

In 1958, Dr. Jarvis published his research in his book *Folk Medicine: A Vermont Doctor's Guide to Good Health*. This publication played an important role in ACV becoming a popular health remedy in America during the rest of the 20th century. However, Jarvis mistakenly attributed ACV's healing powers to what he considered to be its unusually high potassium content. While potassium is certainly a very important mineral necessary for a wide range of healthy functions in the human body, research has subsequently shown that ACV's potassium content is actually not as high as other food sources, and therefore, by itself, the potassium content in ACV cannot fully explain how and why apple cider vinegar is so effective. (You will learn more about this in Chapter 2.)

In addition to Dr. Jarvis, another American health expert played a major role in popularizing apple cider vinegar and a multipurpose health aid during the 20th century. His name was Paul C. Bragg, N.D., Ph.D. Dr. Bragg was born in 1895 and grew up in a farm in Indiana. He was first introduced to the curative powers of ACV by his father. Whenever farm animals were ailing, his father would add ACV to their feed and water to help restore them to health. Every day, he also drank a glass of water to which he would add two teaspoons of apple cider vinegar. As a young boy, curious as to why he did so, Dr. Bragg asked his father about it. His father replied that farming was long and hard work and that his daily ACV drink helped keep him healthy and free from fatigue. For an added burst of energy, his father sometimes also drank a version of switchel.

At the age of 12, Dr. Bragg saved a wealthy man from drowning. As a reward, the man paid for his education at a military academy. There, Bragg's health began to decline, which he later attributed to the unhealthy diet of refined, sugar-laden, and overcooked foods the academy served its young cadets. Eventually, as his health continued to deteriorate, he developed tuberculosis (TB). TB is a potentially fatal disease, and Bragg was sent to a sanitarium in Switzerland to be treated. There, he was surprised to be served a glass of ACV and honey added to water (switchel) every morning to start his day. His daily diet at the healing clinic consisted largely of raw vegetable salads and steamed vegetables, with ACV commonly added to both. Within two years of beginning his treatment there, Bragg was completely cured.

Once he was again healthy, Dr. Bragg dedicated the rest of his life to educating others on the importance of a healthy diet and lifestyle, and about ACV. In the process, he opened the first health food store in the United States and also pioneered the tradition of health lectures across the U.S. He was also the first modern-day health advocate to introduce tomato and pineapple juices, as well as smoothies, to America. In addition, he imported the first hand-juicers to the U.S., introducing the concept of fruit and vegetable juicing to the American public. He also was a prolific author and the creator of his own radio and TV shows focused on "health and happiness."

As Bragg's teachings and influence continued to grow, his expertise as a health expert was sought out by many notable people of his time, including J.C. Penny, Conrad Hilton, real estate developer Delbert Webb, who was also co-owner of the New York Yankees, and Dr. William Scholl, developer of the Dr. Scholl's footwear and foot care brand. Many Hollywood celebrities of the time also were mentored by Dr. Bragg, such as James Cagney, Jane Russell, Gloria Swanson, and Mickey Rooney. Bragg also advised numerous professional and Olympic athletes, as well as mentoring another famous health advocate, Jack LaLanne, who credited Bragg with saving his life at the age of 15 by introducing him to the importance of a healthy diet and lifestyle.

Bragg died in 1976, and today is considered the father of the natural health movement in the U.S. Today, his work is carried on by his daughter (by marriage), Patricia Bragg, who is perhaps the world's foremost proponent of apple cider vinegar for its many health benefits, and the owner of Bragg Live Foods, a producer of its own apple cider vinegar product, as well as many other health products. She is also an author and publisher, and her book *Apple Cider Vinegar: Miracle Health System*, first published in 1990, is largely responsible for the growing popularity ACV has today as a health remedy.

CONCLUSION

As this chapter makes clear, vinegar, in various varieties, has been a part of nearly all cultures around the world for thousands of years, and in each of these cultures vinegar has long been traditionally prized for its health benefits, in addition to its use as a condiment and as a preservative and pickling agent. Given how widely used it is today, with the exception of water, vinegar very well may be the most common and widespread product in the world.

Apple cider vinegar's health properties date back to at least the time of ancient Greece when it was used and recommended by Hippocrates, and since the 1600s ACV has been a staple traditional healing remedy for a wide variety of health conditions. Despite its long and continuous use, however, it was not until the late 20th century that scientists began to research ACV's potential health benefits in earnest. In Chapter 2, you will learn what they are finding out, as well as how and why ACV is such a versatile healer.

2.

How and Why Apple Cider Vinegar Can Improve Your Health

I t's long been said that "an apple a day keeps the doctor away," and with good reason. The health gains associated with apples is due to the abundance of vitamins, minerals, nutrients, and organic compounds that are found in them as you will see in this chapter. This enjoyable fruit is jam-packed with rich phyto-nutrients that are fundamental for optimal health. Specific anti-oxidants in apples have several health bolstering and disease preventing features, and therefore, truly support the motto.

THE APPLE'S HEALTH BENEFITS

Once you take a bite of an apple, you are not only tasting one of nature's most healthful bounty, you are also consuming a rich source of nutrients. Each of these nutrients provides a host of benefits for your body. Each one of the following nutrients will help reduce the risk of disease, such as cancer, cardio-vascular disease, and diabetes.

Minerals

Potassium is a mineral that acts as an electrolyte, meaning that it helps electricity flow through your body. Most potassium in your body is found inside of your cells, but it moves outside of cell walls if necessary, in order to keep fluid steady in and around cells. This process, known as cellular membrane potential, is heavily regulated by your body in order to properly govern and sustain healthy electrical flow for the rhythm of your heartbeat. Potassium is also necessary for proper muscle function and muscle contraction. On average, one medium-sized apple provides about 200 milligrams of potassium.

In addition to potassium, apples contain other important minerals, such as calcium, copper, magnesium, manganese, and zinc, and are a good source of flavonoids. These are a class of plant-based chemicals that have been shown to protect against heart disease, high blood pressure, and certain types of cancer, among other degenerative diseases.

Vitamins

Apples also contain a number of other vital nutrients, including vitamins A, C, and E, all of which act as antioxidants to fight infection and neutralize free radicals that cause inflammation and premature aging in the human body. Apples also supply a number of important B vitamins, including B1 (thiamin), B2 (riboflavin), and B6 (pyridoxine), which work synergistically together to help regulate the body's metabolism and various other vital functions, as well as vitamin K, another antioxidant and anti-inflammatory agent, which is also essential for proper blood clotting and brain and bone health.

Flavonoids

Research has shown that the flavonoids in apples reduce high blood pressure and also regulate blood flow due to their ability to improve endothelial function. The endothelium is a layer of smooth, thin cells that lines the heart and arteries, and helps protect against heart disease in a variety of ways, including preventing substances from sticking to the arterial walls and producing and delivering nitric oxide (NO) to the arteries. NO, which the endothelium produces from the amino acid L-arginine, plays an essential role in keep arteries soft and flexible, allowing them to easily expand so that blood can flow with less effort.

Research has also shown that the flavonoids contained in apples have a preventive effect on certain types of cancer, especially colorectal cancer. Apples' fiber content is also very helpful in this regard. Scientists have found that the more apples a person consumes, the lower his or her risk of colorectal cancer will be. No other fruit has been found to reduce the risk of colorectal cancer to the degree that apples do.

Fiber

Apples are also a good source of pectin, a type of soluble fiber. Research has shown that pectin offers a number of health benefits, including protecting against high cholesterol by lowering LDL (so-called "bad") cholesterol. Pectin has also been found to help reduce high blood sugar levels and to protect against hypertension (high blood pressure). It also helps the body detoxify heavy metals, which can lodge in organs and joints (*see* page 189, Toxic Overload). Pectin does that because of its ability to stick to heavy metals, moving them out of the body via elimination. Pectin further contributes to joint health by stimulating the production of synovial fluid, which helps protect joints and keeps them functioning properly. Among its other benefits, pectin is useful as an aid for weight loss, and can protect against certain forms of cancer, especially prostate cancer.

Most commercially grown apples are among the most pesticide-contaminated produce foods in the U.S. today. Therefore, it is important that you buy and consume apples that are organically grown and harvested.

APPLE CIDER VINEGAR

So, what does all of this have to do with apple cider vinegar? Well, as you might expect, all of the same nutrients contained in apples are also found in ACV. Even the pectin contained in apples becomes a component of ACV.

ACV is also rich in plant-based compounds known as phytochemicals, especially polyphenols. The term *polyphenol* literally means "more than one phenol." Phenols are organic compounds that act as one of Nature's basic chemical building blocks. Polyphenols get their name because they contain more than one phenol group per molecule. Polyphenols are the most abundant class of phenol compounds found in all plants (in this case, apples), and are part of a larger group of compounds known as antioxidants that act to prevent your body's cells and tissues from becoming damaged because of oxidation, a process in which cells and tissues literally begin to "rust out." In many respects polyphenols act as the plants' immune system.

When consumed by humans, polyphenols are very useful in protecting against free radical damage, and scientists are discovering that they provide a variety of other health benefits, as well. One of the main reasons why polyphenols are so important to good health is because they act as catalysts that enable other nutrients to properly do their job. Additionally, unlike most other nutrients, the health benefits polyphenols provide are very broad in scope, including their ability to simultaneously regulate a wide variety of different cell functions.

CV'S KEY INGREDIENT

Because of the supply of nutrients that ACV contains, for many years proponents of using apple cider vinegar for health purposes assumed that it was the nutrients themselves that were responsible for the benefits ACV provides. It turns out, however, that this is not entirely the case. In fact, the typical amount of ACV used to make an apple cider vinegar drink (between one to two teaspoons to one to two tablespoons) contains only a miniscule percentage of these nutrients. Instead, researchers have found that it is not the nutrients themselves that make ACV such a powerful and versatile healing substance, but, rather, the organic acids that apple cider vinegar contains, especially acetic acid.

Acetic Acid

Aside from water, which typically makes up about 95 percent of the content of all vinegars' content, the primary content in vinegar, including apple cider vinegar, is acetic acid. Acetic acid is formed during the fermentation process that produces ACV, and is responsible for ACV's tart flavor as well as its pungent aroma. During that process a group of bacteria known as acetic acid bacteria (*Acetobacter*) or AAB convert the alcohol from which vinegar is derived into acetic acid, as well as other organic acids. During the traditional or slow method of fermentation of vinegar, a nontoxic slime is produced consisting of yeast and AAB. This substance is known as the "mother of vinegar" that you learned about in the Introduction, and its inclusion in ACV products is essential if you hope to get the health benefits that ACV provides).

Although acetic acid is the predominant organic acid produced by the fermentation process that results in ACV, other organic acids are also created during fermentation, including citric acid, as well as various other acids, all of which can also enhance health. Overall, however, it is the acetic acid in ACV that is most important factor for the health benefits ACV provides. This fact has been proven by science.

Scientific Findings

Among the scientific findings about acetic acid is the discovery that it has potent antimicrobial properties, especially against harmful bacteria. Research has shown, for example, that acetic acid is effective at killing E. coli bacteria (*Escherichia coli*), as well as various strains of *Salmonella.* Acetic acid vinegar has also been found to be effective for inhibiting the growth of bacteria on fresh fruits and vegetables. One of the reasons acetic is effective against bacteria is due to its ability to move into the cellular membranes of bacteria, causing them to die off.

Because of this ability, acetic acid has also been shown to also have antiviral properties. In addition, topical application of acetic acid has been shown to be effective for determining the existence of viral infections on the skin. It is for this reason that midwives in indigenous cultures in both Africa and South America use vinegar washes to screen and protect expectant mothers from the human papilloma virus (HPV).

Acetic acid's antimicrobial properties also explain why the use of ACV and other vinegars has proven so effective for helping to heal wounds. The effectiveness comes from the acid's ability to protect against the wounds becoming infected. I find it fascinating that modern science in the 21st century is at last confirming something Hippocrates knew 2500 years ago.

Other research has shown that acetic acid can help protect against high blood sugar (glucose) levels and insulin resistance, making it useful for people who suffer from type 2 diabetes or who are pre-diabetic. Acetic acid achieves these effects due to its anti-glycemic (glucose-reducing) properties. Additional research has also found that acetic acid can help prevent the complete digestion of carbohydrate foods, including complex carbohydrates to further prevent blood sugar and insulin spikes.

Related research has also found that acetic acid can offer benefits for people who are overweight or obese because of its anti-glycemic effects, as well as its ability to produce feelings of satiety (feeling full) if taken prior to and during meals. This, in turn, can lead to reduced food consumption at meals, resulting in a lower intake of calories.

Another important benefit of acetic acid lies in its ability to lower blood levels of LDL ("bad") cholesterol and protect against elevated triglycerides. Both high LDL cholesterol and elevated triglycerides levels are markers for heart disease, meaning that acetic acid can be beneficial for protecting against our nation's number one killer. Acetic acid compounds have also been demonstrated to protect against high blood pressure (hypertension) by helping to prevent constriction of the arteries and other blood vessels. This was shown in studies that found that acetic acid reduces the activity of the compounds renin and plasma aldosterone, both of which are associated with blood vessel constriction.

I will discuss the studies that have confirmed the above findings about acetic acid in the appropriate disease conditions mentioned in Part Two of this book. For now, let me conclude this chapter by mentioning two other important benefits of acetic acid, as well as the various other organic acids that apple cider vinegar contains.

The first has to do with the ability of acetic acid and other organic acids to stimulate the growth of healthy flora in the gastrointestinal tract. In this regard, the acids act in much the same way as probiotics, such as *Lactobacillus* and *Bifidobacterium* do. However, the organic acids contained in ACV are not probiotics. Rather, they can more accurately be likened to *prebiotics.*

The difference between probiotics and prebiotics is simple. Probiotics are themselves types of healthy flora which, when consumed, add to the GI tract's population of healthy bacteria. Prebiotics, on the other hand, stimulate the further growth of health flora that is already present in the GI tract, similar to the way fertilizers stimulate the growth of plants. Research has long demonstrated that an abundant supply of health flora in the GI tract is essential for overall gastrointestinal function, as well as for proper functioning of the immune system.

A second significant benefit of ACV's organic acids is also related to the GI tract. It has to do with the acids' ability to improve your body's ability to more fully absorb and make use of nutrients, including not only the nutrients that ACV itself contains, but, far more importantly, the wide array of nutrients that you consume each day in your food. In this respect, ACV's organic acids act in much the same way that enzymes do, helping your body to more easily break down food, and better assimilate and metabolize nutrients. This is important, because if your body is unable to efficiently assimilate and make use of the nutrients contained in your food the end result is nutritional deficiencies that negatively impact the literally hundreds of vital functions your body constantly performs.

CONCLUSION

Now that you have a better understanding of just how and why apple cider vinegar can provide so many health benefits, let's turn our attention to what you must know in order to choose and use an apple cider vinegar product so that you can be sure of obtaining the full range of health benefits ACV can provide. That is the focus of the next chapter.

3.

Guidelines for Choosing an Apple Cider Vinegar Product

In order to obtain the full range of health benefits that apple cider provides, it is essential that you know what to look for when choosing an ACV product, and how to best use it once you have selected it. This chapter explains how to do so.

The first step in using apple cider vinegar is to know what to look for when you purchase an ACV product. There are three key questions to keep in mind before you do so:

- Is the apple cider vinegar filtered or unfiltered?

- Is it pasteurized or unpasteurized (raw)?

- Does it contain "the mother?"

When it comes to your health, the most effective type of apple cider vinegar should be filtered, unpasteurized, and most definitely contain "the mother." Let me explain.

WHY YOU WANT TO AVOID FILTERED, PASTEURIZED ACV PRODUCTS

Most commercially available apple cider vinegar products that you will find at your local grocery store are filtered and pasteurized, rather than unfiltered and unpasteurized. If you are simply using ACV as a flavoring agent or as a home cleaning aid (all vinegars have many uses as a nontoxic home cleanser), then filtered, pasteurized ACV products are fine. However, if you want to use ACV to help improve your health, you need to look for an unfiltered, unpasteurized ACV product.

The reason for this is simple. When ACV is filtered (processed or distilled), the "mother of vinegar" and the potent combination of acetic and other organic acids that ACV naturally contains are removed before the vinegar is bottled for sale. That means that filtered ACV will not supply you with these important organic compounds which, as you learned in Chapter 2, are the primary reason why ACV in its natural state can be so effective for so many health-related purposes.

Pasteurized vs Unpasteurized ACV

Unpasteurized ACV simply means that it is raw or in its pure, natural, unadulterated state. In other words, it has not been filtered, heated, or otherwise refined in any way, nor has it been subject to any sort of other processing, and nothing else has been added to it. Pasteurized ACV, on the other hand, has been sterilized (that is how pasteurization occurs), either by being exposed to high heat or through a process of irradiation.

The purpose of pasteurization is to kill off potentially harmful bacteria. Properly prepared unfiltered and unpasteurized ACV, however, does not contain harmful bacteria, meaning that when it is pasteurized, the rich supply of healthy bacteria ACV is killed off instead. As a result, like filtered ACV, ACV that has been pasteurized is incapable of providing the same degree of health benefits that unpasteurized ACV supplies.

Another important distinction between pasteurized and unpasteurized ACV is that unpasteurized apple cider vinegar is most often produced from organic apples, whereas pasteurized ACV is usually made from nonorganic apples. This is important, because nonorganic, commercially grown and harvested apples in the United States have consistently ranked as high as second among the top 12 types of produce with the highest content of harmful pesticides, according to the annual listing of the Environmental Working Groups "Dirty Dozen" report.

Filtered vs Unfliltered

You can easily distinguish between filtered, pasteurized and unfiltered, unpasteurized ACV by looking at the bottle. Filtered ACV will be clear throughout, with no trace of sediment in the bottle, while unfiltered ACV will appear cloudy, with sediment from "the mother" being clearly visible, often at the bottom of the bottle. The product label will also tell you what type of ACV the bottle contains. You want to choose an ACV product that the label clearly states is raw or unfiltered, organic, unpasteurized, and contains "the mother." Such ACV products are readily available in health food stores, and can increasingly be found in the organic food aisles of grocery stores. I've also included a listing of manufacturers of this type of ACV in the Resources section.

THE IMPORTANCE OF "THE MOTHER"

As I mentioned, the health benefits you wish to obtain from using apple cider vinegar will only be available to you if your chosen ACV product contains "the mother of vinegar" because it is this substance that contains the rich supply of concentrated organic acids, enzymes, and nutrients that give ACV its various health-enhancing properties.

The "mother of vinegar" gets its name because it is what the French merchants who developed the Orleans method of vinegar production relied upon when they discovered how to continuously produce vinegar. As you learned in Chapter 1, as the vinegar was produced, approximately 15 percent of it was left behind in each cask. This remaining vinegar became known as "the mother" vinegar due to the concentrated bacteria it contained (AAB, which you learned about in Chapter 2). Small amounts of the AAB-rich mother vinegar were then added to new barrels of the wine which the Orleans merchants used to quick start the production of additional batches of vinegar. It is the mother of vinegar with its culture of beneficial bacteria that turns regular apple cider into vinegar in the first place

In appearance, "mother of vinegar" has a slime-like quality due to the gummy, jelly-like layer of film that characterizes it. This film typically forms on the top of apple cider vinegar as it is being produced, giving ACV a cloudy appearance. Often the film looks to be composed of wisps, giving it the appearance of spider webs. In actuality, the "mother of vinegar" is composed of cellulose combined with AAB. During each new process of fermentation the AAB in the "mother of vinegar" combines with oxygen to create new batches of vinegar and to produce acetic acid and the various other organic acids that ACV contains.

Despite the health benefits apple cider vinegar with "the mother" supplies, these days it is becoming harder to find natural vinegars containing "the mother" on the grocery store shelf. Largely due to its appearance which, to those who are not aware of "the mother's" benefits, may not look appealing, most commercial manufacturers of ACV today prefer to pasteurize, filter, and distill apple cider vinegar to get rid of "the mother." Fortunately, though, raw, unfiltered apple cider vinegar containing "the mother" is what is sold in most health food stores You can also find suppliers online (*see* Resources).

BEWARE OF ACV SUPPLEMENTS— CAPSULES AND TABLETS

Because of the growing awareness of apple cider vinegar's health benefits, a number of nutritional supplement companies have started to produce and sell apple cider vinegar supplements in the form of tablets and capsule. Such products can be found in many health food stores, and often in the vitamin aisles of grocery and drugstores. The makers of such products will often claim that their capsules or tablets supply the same benefits of a glass of liquid apple cider vinegar in water, and that they are easier and more convenient to use. Despite such claims, I do not recommend them.

There are a number of reasons why I caution against the use of ACV supplements. First, unlike liquid apple cider vinegar, as well as acetic acid solutions, both of which are now beginning to be researched by scientists for their health benefits and safety, no such research exists for ACV supplements. Moreover, it can sometimes be difficult to know the manufacturing standards to which supplement companies adhere. Some companies, unfortunately, in order to maximize their profits, follow less than stringent manufacturing policies.

Another concern has to do with the quality or lack thereof of the ingredients used in the production of nutritional supplements. Again for cost-cutting purposes, certain companies use low-grade ingredients. In addition, unlike apple cider vinegar itself, ACV supplements often contain fillers, including, in some cases, unhealthy artificial flavors. Research has also found that the amount of each nutrient listed on supplement labels are not always accurate, with the supplements often containing far less of the ingredients than what is claimed in the labeling.

The above issues exist because, in the United States, the nutritional supplement industry is not regulated by the Food and Drug Administration (FDA) and other government regulatory agencies to the same degree that food producers are. Since apple cider vinegar is a food product, you can have greater assurance that it contains precisely what the product label says it contains, in the concentrations by volume listed on the label and with no other unlisted additives.

Finally, as you learned above, when consumed orally in its liquid form, ACV should always be diluted with a much greater volume of water. ACV supplements, on the other hand, are not diluted in this way, increasing their risk that they may be harmful. In fact, there has been at least one reported case of an ACV supplement causing damage to a person's throat (specifically her esophagus), when an ACV tablet she consumed unexpectedly became stuck in her throat, causing serious esophageal damage before it could be dislodged. Therefore, just as, ideally, it is better to obtain all of the nutrients your body needs from the foods and beverages you consume, I recommend that you consume apple cider vinegar the way healers throughout history have used it—in its liquid form diluted in water.

HOW TO USE APPLE CIDER VINEGAR

Now that you know what to look for when selecting an apple cider vinegar product, let's explore the guidelines for its use. As you will learn in more detail in Part Two, ACV can be used both topically and orally. You will find instructions for how to use ACV topically in the applicable health conditions sections covered in Part Two. This chapter focuses on how to use it orally.

The typical oral recommended dose of apple cider vinegar is one tablespoon of ACV added to a glass of 8 to 12 ounces of pure, filtered water (it is not a good idea to drink unfiltered tap water because of the contaminants most municipal tap water contains), taken one to three times a day, ideally at least 20 minutes before meals. However, if you are unused to apple cider vinegar drinks, ACV's tart, bitter taste may take a bit of time to get used to. Therefore, it may be more advisable to start slow, using no more than one to two teaspoons of ACV added to a single glass of pure, unfiltered water per day. Over time, you can then increase your dosage to one to two tablespoons and drink one or more glasses per day, depending on your needs and comfort level.

Caution: Because of its acidic nature, it is important to remember that apple cider vinegar *must always be diluted in water before being consumed.* Consumed by itself, ACV can cause a burning sensation in your mouth and throat, and possibly even cause inflammation or irritation of throat tissue. Undiluted ACV can also soften and damage tooth enamel. In fact, if you have sensitive teeth, you might want to drink even fully diluted ACV through a straw to minimize contact between your ACV drink and your teeth.

STORAGE AND PACKAGING

Nearly all varieties of apple cider vinegar (both raw, unfiltered, and unpasteurized products and filtered, pasteurized versions) are sold in glass bottles, although some companies use plastic containers as well. Glass bottles are the preferable option, both because they provide a clearer view of their contents, and, more importantly, because plastic bottles may contain harmful chemicals that can potentially leach into the vinegar over time. However, some reputable companies that sell raw, organic, unpasteurized apple cider vinegar sometimes do offer ACV in plastic containers. Typically, they do so for ACV sold in higher volume (quart and half-gallon sizes). If you intend to use a lot of apple cider vinegar, then this can be a more economical choice. If you have them handy, you can also pour the ACV into glass bottles once you bring your purchase home, making sure to cap the bottles tightly after you fill them up.

Since all types of vinegar, including ACV, act as natural preservatives, storing apple cider vinegar requires no special care. For best results, make sure you tightly reseal the cap on the bottle after each use, and although ACV does not require refrigeration (although you can refrigerate it if you like), it is advisable to keep bottles of ACV away from sunlight. Also be sure to use apple cider vinegar before its expiration date, which you can find on the product label.

SOME FURTHER CAUTIONS ABOUT USING ACV

Although apple cider vinegar has a long, established record of being safe to use both orally and topically, like nearly everything else, using too much of it can still pose certain possible health risks. Therefore, as with any other addition to your daily health routine, I strongly recommend that you inform your doctor before you begin consuming ACV drinks in case he or she has any precautions you may need to know about. This is especially true if you are using any prescription medications (check the labels of your medications or ask your doctor). In particular, diabetics who are on insulin or other diabetes drugs should always use ACV with caution, as ACV can potentially interfere with such drugs. People who are on medications to lower potassium levels, such as diuretic drugs, should also consult with their physicians before using ACV drinks because of the potassium ACV contains. People who suffer from or who are at risk for osteoporosis (bone loss) are also advised to consult with a physician before beginning ACV use. Finally, if you are pregnant or a nursing mother you should also speak with your doctor because residues of ACV, after it is consumed, may prove irritating to your developing fetus and infant child.

If you follow the above recommendations for taking ACV orally, you should experience no problems. However, there are certain side effects that can occur with overconsumption of ACV, including, as I mentioned above, irritation or inflammation of throat tissues and softening of or damage to tooth enamel.

Some people may also experience temporary stomach upset if they are unused to ACV, especially if their stomachs are already producing robust levels of hydrochloric acid (HCl).(Most people in the U.S., especially as they age, are actually deficient in HCl production). If a stomach ache occurs, you can usually quickly alleviate it by drinking more pure, unfiltered water without ACV. To prevent further flare-ups, you can reduce the amount of ACV you use in your ACV drinks. Adding a quarter teaspoon of pure (non-aluminum-containing) baking soda to your ACV drink can also be helpful because of baking soda's alkalizing properties and ability to neutralize acidity.

Because ACV drinks help your body to cleanse and detoxify, some people may also experience temporary flare-ups of skin conditions. Your skin is your body's largest organ of detoxification, and such skin conditions can often be signs that toxins are moving out of your body. If such eruptions are triggered by ACV, they will usually pass quickly. If they don't, stop consuming ACV drinks and, if necessary, consult with your doctor or a dermatologist.

CONCLUSION

By following the above guidelines and sensible precautions, you can rest assured that you are ready to begin your journey of discovery of how apple cider vinegar can help you address your specific health concerns. First, though, for those of you who are so inclined, I'd like to tell you how you can easily and inexpensively make your own homemade supply of apple cider vinegar. To find out, turn to Chapter 4.

4.

How to Make Your Own Apple Cider Vinegar

Store-bought, raw, organic, unpasteurized apple cider vinegar is inexpensive, with each serving costing only pennies. It is also relatively easy to find, especially at health food stores. Still, some people prefer to make their own apple cider vinegar at home. If the thought of doing so appeals to you, this chapter is for you.

GETTING STARTED

Producing apple cider vinegar at home is relatively easy and can be a fun, educational experience for your family. No special equipment is required. Here is all you will need to get started:

- 2 clean wide mouth glass containers, such as a mason jar
- 1 or more small mouth glass container(s), with lid(s)
- A clean cotton or cheese cloth to be used as a covering
- An additional cheese cloth to be used as a strainer
- A rubber band
- Organic apples (Apples harvested in the fall are best)
- Apple scraps (cores and peels) can also be used
- 2 tablespoons to 1 cup or pure cane sugar or raw, organic honey (depending on how much ACV you wish to make at one time)
- Pure, filtered or distilled water

Once you have the equipment and ingredients, you are ready for *stage one:*

1. First make sure the open mouth glass container is clean and dry.
2. Next, thoroughly wash three to ten medium-sized apples, and then cut them into chunks, removing the stems and, if you wish, the seeds (apple

seeds are actually healthy to eat, and you can include them if you wish). If you are using scraps instead of apples to start, double the amount of cores.

3. Set the apple chunks or scraps in the air, allowing them to brown, which will happen very quickly.

4. Once the chunks or scraps turn brown, place them in the open mouth container. Regardless of the size container you use, the apples should fill at least half of the container. If not, continue to add more apple chunks or scraps until they do.

5. Then add enough room temperature water until the apples or apple scraps are completely submerged. I recommend using distilled water, if you have it, otherwise pure, filtered water is fine. Once the water is added, the entire mixture should fill nearly all of the container, leaving only a few inches of space at the top. This space is necessary so that there is enough oxygen to interact with the finished mixture, creating the process of fermentation. **Important:** The apples or scraps must be completely covered by water to prevent mold growth.

6. Next add in either the pure cane sugar or raw, organic honey and stir thoroughly until it entirely dissolves.

7. Once the mixture is complete, cover the glass container lid with clean cotton or cheese cloth, securing it over the lid with a rubber band. (If you are using a cheese cloth, you may need to double it up because you do not want it to be too porous. Too much porosity will interfere with the fermentation process.)

8. Once the container is covered and sealed with the cloth, set the container in a cupboard or closet shelf or on a countertop away from sunlight, where it will remain for two to three weeks, depending on how long it needs to fully ferment. During this time, gently stir the mixture once or twice each day.

It is during this two to three week process that the mixture will ferment to turn into a version of hard apple cider. You will notice this occurring by the presence of small bubbles in the water. This is a sign that the sugar or honey, as it interacts with the oxygen in the container, is fermenting the apple mixture. As this process occurs, you will also begin to notice the pleasant aroma of apple cider as it forms.

For most of the time that you set the container aside, the apple chunks or scraps you used will continue to float within it. Eventually, though, the apples will begin to settle to the bottom of the container. Once they fully do so, you will know that the mixture has fully turned into hard apple cider. When that happens, you are ready for stage two—the transformation of the apple cider mixture into apple cider vinegar.

Sometimes the apple mixture may not fully settle to the bottom before the mixture fully turns into cider. To be sure, you can taste the mixture from time to time. Once it is ready, you can be sure that you will be able to taste it.

Stage two is very easy to prepare:

1. Simply strain the mixture in the first container through a double folded cheese cloth into the second, same-sized glass container (be sure that it is clean), discarding the solid apple remains.

2. Then cover the second container with the original clean cotton or cheese cloth, securing it over the lid with the rubber band.

3. Once you finish, set the second container aside for another four to six weeks, once again keeping the container from being exposed to direct sunlight. There is no need to stir the mixture during this second stage.

It is during this time that the alcohol produced from the fermentation of the original mixture into cider will further ferment and be transformed into the acetic acid and other organic acids that will change the mixture into apple cider vinegar. As it does so, you will begin to notice a small amount of sediment forming on the bottom of the clear mixture in the new container. Around the same time, wispy strands of additional sediment will begin forming at the top of the mixture. The appearance of these sediment strands is a sign that "the mother of vinegar" is being produced. Once these strands appear, usually within the first three weeks, you can begin to taste test the mixture until you are satisfied that it tastes like apple cider vinegar. Once it has the correct level of vinegar taste that you are pleased with, strain the mixture one more time, pouring it into one or more small mouth glass bottles, and seal the bottle or bottles with a lid to use as you desire. Voila! You have now produced your first batch of raw, organic apple cider vinegar.

A Few Additional Tips

During both stages of the fermentation process, the glass containers should be kept in a temperature that never drops below 60 degrees Fahrenheit or above 80 degrees Fahrenheit.

If after 4 to 6 weeks, the vinegary taste of the mixture still isn't quite strong enough for you, you can set it aside for another week and then taste it again. If it still doesn't taste as it should, throw the mixture out and try again. Conversely, if you find that you have left the mixture too long and its vinegary taste is too strong, simply dilute it with some more pure, filtered or distilled water to a level of acidity that best agrees with you.

APPLE CIDER VINEGAR DRINK RECIPES

As you learned in Chapter 3, a basic apple cider vinegar tonic can be prepared simply by adding between one to two teaspoons to one to two tablespoons of ACV to an 8 to 12 ounce glass of pure, filtered water.

If you prefer to give your ACV drink an added zest, here are a few recipes you can try, using either your homemade or store-bought apple cider vinegar.

■ Lemony-Cinnamon ACV

In addition to ACV and water, add one to two tablespoons of fresh-squeezed lemon juice, plus a dash or two of cinnamon powder to the drink, then stir thoroughly.

■ ACV With Green Tea

Like apple cider vinegar, green tea offers many health benefits. Combining ACV with green tea can enhance the energizing effects of both ingredients. To do so, simply bring water to a boil, then pour some of it into a cup. Add a green tea bag (be sure the green tea you use is organic) to the water and let it steep for 10 to 15 minutes. Then add a teaspoon of ACV. For added flavor, you can also add a teaspoon of honey. This is a particularly refreshing drink to start your morning with, especially in winter, and is an excellent substitute for coffee.

■ ACV "Soda"

This drink is a healthy alternative for soda. Simply add one tablespoon of ACV to a glass of mineral or sparkling water, along with a teaspoon of honey, and stir thoroughly.

There are many other fun and delicious ways of combining apple cider vinegar with other healthy ingredients to create a variety of other refreshing ACV drinks. I encourage you to experiment on your own to discover the varieties you most enjoy.

HOW TO MAKE YOUR OWN SWITCHEL DRINKS

In Chapter 1, you learned about switchel, an ACV-based tonic that became popular in the United States, starting in the 1700s. Like apple cider vinegar itself, switchel drinks are very easy to make at home, and require far less time. Once you have produced your home batch of ACV (you can also use store-bought ACV, of course), here are some basic switchel recipes you can try.

■ Basic Switchel Recipe

The basic switchel recipe consists of only four ingredients: water, ACV, honey, and ginger powder. To make more than one serving, combine half a cup of ACV with half a cup of raw, organic honey (you can use less honey if you prefer a more tart flavor) and mix them thoroughly together (you may wish to warm the honey first, to make mixing easier). Once you are done, add the mixture to 2 quarts of water, along with a tablespoon of ginger powder, and stir everything together. Provides eight to ten servings (keep unused portions refrigerated).

Variations

As a variation to this recipe, you can also add a quarter cup of blackstrap molasses to the honey and ACV before adding all three to the water. Black strap molasses is a rich source of calcium, magnesium, iron, and potassium, as well as vitamin B6, and acts as a natural energizing agent, as well as an antioxidant. Including it in your switchel drink will boost the health benefits switchel can provide.

To enhance the flavor of your switchel drink, you can add a sprig of mint to each glass. Some recipes also suggest adding a handful of fresh berries to switchel after it is prepared, and then to let everything sit for 20 to 30 minutes, so that the berry flavors can be absorbed. You can also combine the mint with the berries to make an even zestier drink.

CONCLUSION

Whether you choose to make your own apple cider vinegar at home, or prefer to simply buy ACV at the store, I hope that you will begin to try the above ACV and switchel drink recipes and make the drinks a part of your daily routine because of the boosts they can give to your health and energy levels.

Now that you know how to use apple cider vinegar, and how to make it on your own if you are so inclined, no doubt you are now ready to explore the many ways that ACV acts as a natural healer. That is the focus of Part Two. First, though, let's take a look at how you can take the next step to creating an improved overall healthy lifestyle.

5.

Taking the Next Steps to Better Health

For all of the health benefits apple cider vinegar provides, it would be a mistake to think that simply using it on a regular basis is all you need to do to improve your health. While using ACV regular certainly will supply you with a variety health benefits, neither it nor any other type of health product, by itself, is capable of providing you with lasting optimal health.

As a culture, when it comes to our health, most people seek "quick fix" solutions. Far too often we are prone to place our hopes on a single "magic" ingredient or therapy that can make all of our health problems disappear. In reality, such quick fix, magical solutions do not exist. Your health, like everything else that truly matters in your life, depends on what you do each and every day. As the ancient Greek philosopher Aristotle taught, we become what our habits make us. Simply put, bad habits lead to bad results; good habits lead to good outcomes. This is especially true when it comes to health and disease. If you desire to be truly healthy, you need to adopt healthy habits that you follow each and every day.

There are many things you can do to try and improve your health, but the best approach for doing so is one that focuses on the following key pillars, each of which is essential for creating a solid foundation that can best insure you will live a long, healthy life with abundant energy. These key pillars are a healthy diet, proper hydration, regular exercise, proper and adequate sleep, and stress management. The rest of this chapter provides guidelines you can follow for each of them.

A HEALTHY DIET

It should go without saying that a healthy diet is a vital cornerstone of optimal health. Unfortunately, the standard American diet, aptly abbreviated as SAD, is anything but healthy. In fact, it is downright dangerous to your health, consisting as it does of numerous unhealthy fats, sugars, food additives, and other suspect ingredients, while being severely deficient in the many vitamins, minerals, and other nutrients that your body needs to function properly.

Why is diet so important to your health? Because the foods you eat supply the fuel your body needs—in the form of vitamins, minerals, enzymes, amino acids, essential fatty acids, and other nutrients—to perform its thousands of daily functions. The better your fuel supply (the foods you eat) is, the better able your body is to generate energy, repair itself, and resist invading pathogens. Conversely, eating poorly diminishes your body's ability to maintain optimum functioning.

Fortunately, following a healthy diet is not difficult. In fact, it's quite easy to do once you know how to do so. Here are some important general guidelines to get you started. They have long been recommended by nutritionally oriented physicians and many health organizations, yet they continued to be ignored by tens of millions of Americans, a fact that goes a long way toward explaining our nation's current healthcare crisis. Given that healthy diet alone can greatly reduce your risk of serious health conditions, including our nation's two top killers—heart disease and cancer—I cannot overstate how important these guidelines can be to your health.

Eat Lots of Fresh Fruits and Vegetables

A plentiful supply of fresh fruits and vegetables needs to be a staple of your daily diet. These food groups are rich with vital nutrients and enzymes and also high in fiber. Be sure to eat at least a portion of your daily vegetable intake raw, since high temperatures from cooking can destroy their nutrient and enzyme content. Lightly steaming vegetables is another healthy cooking alternative.

Overall, try to eat at least 7 to 10 servings of fruits and vegetables every day. Also be sure to eat from a wide variety of fruits and vegetables to help ensure you obtain a broad spectrum of nutrients. I find one of the easiest ways to eat a variety of vegetables is by including them in salads topped with a dressing of extra virgin olive oil, apple cider vinegar, and seasonings to taste.

Eat a Variety of Foods

Many people today are deficient in essential nutrients because they routinely eat a limited variety of foods meal after meal. Not only does such "diet monotony" limit nutrient intake, it also can lead to food allergies and sensitivities, both of which are common, yet frequently undiagnosed, health conditions. By eating a wide variety of foods, you have a much better likelihood of avoiding such conditions, and can also increase your nutrient intake.

Eat Organic Foods

Whenever possible, try to eat organic foods. Organic fruits and vegetables have been shown to have a higher nutrient content, compared to non-organic produce, and are also free of harmful pesticides, preservatives, and other chemicals used to grow non-organic, commercial food crops. Similarly, your meat and poultry food choices should ideally be free-range and free of the hormones and antibiotics that are commonly given to commercially-harvested animal products.

Include Essential Fatty Acids

Contrary to popular belief, all of us require a certain amount of fat in our diet. Fats act as your body's energy reserves, and serve as a primary form of insulation, helping to maintain normal body temperature. In addition, fats assist in transporting oxygen, help in the absorption of fat-soluble vitamins, and act as natural anti-inflammatory agents. Fats also help nourish the skin, nerves, and mucous membranes. The best sources of fat in the diet are essential fatty acids (EFAs), particularly omega-3s and omega-6s. Many people have an excess of omega-6s in their diet, compared to omega-3s, so taking care to ensure a proper balance between the two is important. Good sources of omega-3 EFAs include herring, mackerel, sardines, wild-caught salmon, wild game, flaxseed and flaxseed oil, walnuts, and pumpkin seeds.

You should also include some saturated fat in your diet because, contrary to popular belief, such fats are also good for you. Until recently, saturated fats, found in red meats, milk, butter, cheese and other dairy products, were also linked to health problems, and recommended to be consumed sparingly. New evidence, however, suggests that the health risks of saturated fat consumption have been overstated, and that moderate saturated fat consumption is actually healthy. So don't worry about treating yourself to such foods, just take care not to overdo it.

Eat Plenty of Fiber

The standard American diet supplies no more than a third (and often even less) of the amount of fiber necessary for optimum health. Yet research shows that a high fiber diet is closely associated with lower incidences of heart disease, high blood pressure, certain types of cancer (especially colon and rectal cancer), diabetes, constipation, hemorrhoids, gall bladder disease, and gastrointestinal conditions, such as colitis and diverticulitis. Good sources of fiber include fruits, vegetables, bran, rolled oats, brown rice, and other complex carbohydrates.

Eliminate "Junk" Foods

This should go without saying. Simply put, these foods are unhealthy and, when eaten on a regular basis, will inevitably lead to disease. Junk foods are so named because they are overloaded with chemicals, colorings, trans-fats, excess sugars, and other additives that are bad for our health. Moreover, they are typically high in calories and low in nutrient content. If you truly are committed to your health, you will avoid eating such foods altogether.

Avoid Simple Sugars and Refined Carbohydrates

The average American consumes 150 pounds of simple or refined sugar each and every year. This is the equivalent of more than 40 teaspoons of sugar a day, which goes a long way towards explaining why, as a nation, we are so sick. Sugar's many harmful effects include increasing the risk of heart disease, weakening the immune system and increasing susceptibility to infection, stimulating excessive insulin production, increasing the production of harmful triglycerides, diminishing mental function, increasing feelings of anxiety and depression, increasing the risk of cancer, and increasing systemic yeast overgrowth (candidiasis).

To effectively eliminate sugar from your diet, it is important that you read food labels, since sugar is a common ingredient in packaged foods in the forms of fructose, sucrose, corn syrup, lactose, and maltose. In general, foods that are canned, processed, or cured are also likely to be high in sugar. Healthy sugar substitutes include raw, organic honey, stevia, and, eaten sparingly, dark chocolate.

Refined carbohydrates act in much the same way that sugar does when consumed and metabolized in your body. Therefore, they should be avoided altogether. Refined, or simple, carbohydrates include white breads, pastas made from white flour, instant mashed potatoes, white rice, chips, and sugar laden commercial cereals. The most common health risks when these foods are consumed on a regular basis are excessive insulin production, excessive fat storage, and elevated blood sugar levels. Obesity and diabetes are two of the most serious health conditions directly linked to frequent consumption of these foods.

Eliminate Unhealthy Fats

As I mentioned above, certain fats are essential for good health. Unfortunately, many of us, instead of eating foods rich in healthy fats, consume harmful fats such as trans-fatty acids and hydrogenated fats, both of which have been linked to a host of disease conditions, including arteriosclerosis, heart attack, angina, cancer, kidney failure, and obesity. Trans-fatty acids and hydrogenated fats are commonly found in margarine, cooking fats, commercial peanut butter, commercial cereals, and packaged foods.

Minimize Caffeine

It is estimated that more than half of all Americans are addicted to caffeine, primarily through drinking coffee. While caffeine in moderation (one to two cups of coffee per day) is not only harmless, but provides a variety of health benefits, too much regular caffeine consumption can contribute to a wide range of health problems, and can decrease platelet stickiness, thus interfering with the blood clotting process. It can also cause loss of calcium in the body, thereby disrupting acid-alkaline (pH) balance. If you enjoy drinking coffee, we recommend organic blends.

If you rely on coffee or other caffeine drinks to give you a boost of energy during the day, you may find that substituting with the apple cider vinegar and switchel drinks covered in Chapter 4 will provide you with the same benefits without any of the health risks excess caffeine intake can trigger.

Minimize, But Don't Eliminate, Your Salt Intake

Salt is another ingredient that is far too prevalent in the standard American diet. However, a certain amount of salt is required by your body in order to carry out its many functions. It's when we consume too much salt that health problems can arise. When salt intake is excessive, water is drawn into the bloodstream, increasing blood volume. This, in turn, can increase blood pressure levels, and also interfere with the ability of the body's lymphatic system to eliminate waste matter from the cells.

Additionally, many brands of commercial salt lack iodine (which is essential for proper thyroid function) and other essential trace minerals that are found in salt in its natural state. Therefore, I recommend that, when you do use salt, you choose sea or Celtic salt, both of which are rich in such co-factor minerals.

PROPER HYDRATION— YOUR BODY'S MANY NEEDS FOR WATER

One of the easiest and most powerful things you can do for your health is to be sure and drink adequate amounts of pure, filtered water each and every day.

That fact shouldn't be surprising. After all, approximately 70 to 75 percent of your body is composed of water. (In the bodies of babies, water composition is closer to 80 percent.) Because this is so, water is the medium through which all of your body functions occur.

Despite this fact, most doctors and health practitioners rarely consider whether or not their patients are meeting their daily water requirements. This is one of the reasons that so many people today *aren't* drinking enough water each day. Making matters worse, the standard American diet that most people follow these days further interferes with the numerous functions that water helps your body perform. The end result is that many people are today chronically dehydrated and they don't even know it.

Water's Health Benefits

Water's numerous health benefits were clearly established by the late Dr. Fereydoon Batmanghelidj, who was recognized as the world's foremost authority on the relationship between water and health, and dehydration and disease. I had the pleasure of meeting Dr. Batman, as he liked to be called, and it is because of his research that he shared with me that I now know how important it is to keep our bodies properly hydrated.

Dr. Batmanghelidj spent the last decades of his life exclusively studying and documenting how powerful water can be as a healing tool. He maintained that the primary cause of many illnesses was chronic dehydration, and his findings are reported in his books *Your Body's Many Cries for Water* and *You're Not Sick, You're Thirsty!* As he explained in his writings, since water is the medium that regulates all body functions, when we fail to provide our bodies with all of the water it requires each day to remain properly hydrated, over time many of our bodily functions become compromised and eventually damage and disease take hold.

Based on his research, Dr. Batmanghelidj became convinced that nearly everyone in the United States suffers from chronic, low-grade dehydration. His research also demonstrated that chronic, low-grade dehydration plays a primary role in many of the chronic diseases that beset our nation today. More importantly, he found that in many cases simply restoring the body to a properly hydrated state was enough to reverse these health conditions or, at the very least, reduce their symptoms. Yet, despite publishing his research and findings in medical journals, both in the US and around the world, his work continues to be ignored by the medical profession. As a result, few people today understand the powerful positive difference that water can make in their health. Water is also essential for:

- Enhancing immune function, especially in bone marrow, where immune cells are formed
- Increasing the ability and efficiency of oxygen collection in the lungs by red blood cells
- Maintaining proper elimination and preventing constipation
- Stabilizing and maintaining the health of the discs of the spine
- Maintaining the health of the heart and overall cardiovascular system

- Enhancing overall brain function (85 percent of your brain is composed of water)
- Maintaining proper metabolism and digestion
- Maintaining proper kidney and urinary function
- Maintaining proper liver function
- Maintaining proper regulation of body temperature via perspiration
- Maintaining proper joint lubrication and muscle function
- Maintaining healthy respiratory function
- Maintaining proper function of the lymphatic system and the elimination of waste products via urine
- Maintaining healthy functioning of the immune system
- Maintaining healthy skin
- Maintaining proper delivery of oxygen into the cells and the elimination of cellular wastes
- Maintaining proper function of the body's "heating" and "cooling" systems
- Maintaining proper production of your body's hormones and neurotransmitters.

Water Transports Oxygen

In addition to being essential for regulating all of your body's functions, water is also necessary for transporting oxygen to your body's cells, tissues, and organs. When you fail to drink enough water your body starts to become deprived of the oxygen it needs. That's because oxygen, as it enters your body, is dissolved in water and then transported to all of your body's cells, tissues, and organs. When you are dehydrated, this process is impeded, leaving you oxygen deficient.

Water Breaks Down the Food You Eat

Your body also uses water to break down the food you eat into smaller particles. This process, in turn, enables the vitamins, minerals, and other vital nutrients foods contain to be metabolized and assimilated, while at the same time enabling food's unnecessary byproducts, or waste, to be eliminated.

Water as a Primary Source of Energy

Water, along with oxygen, is also one of your body's primary sources of energy. It literally generates electrical and magnetic energy inside each and every one of your body's trillions upon trillions of cells. This is especially important for healthy brain function, since the brain depends on an adequate water supply to operate.

Water Acts as a Bonding Substance

In addition, water also acts as a bonding substance that enables your cells to maintain their proper structure. Without enough water, cell structure cannot be properly maintained, leading to a loss of structural integrity and, eventually, disease.

Water Prevents Damage and Aids in Repair of Your DNA

Water also helps to prevent your body's DNA from being damaged and aids in its ability to repair itself. DNA (deoxyribonucleic acid) contains your genetic code and is found within each of your body's cells, keeping them healthy and properly functioning. When DNA becomes damaged it can cause cells to behave abnormally. Abnormal DNA is a known cause of cancer, as well as various other disease conditions. This means that, by drinking enough water each day, you can literally improve your resistance to cancer.

Are You Dehydrated?

Most people assume they simply need to pay attention to whether or not they feel thirsty to know if they need to drink more water. They wait until their mouths become dry before thinking about drinking something. However, as Dr. Batmangheldij's research repeatedly showed, a dry mouth is actually the last outward sign that your body is dehydrated. That's because feelings of thirst don't develop until long after your body's water supply has fallen well below the level needed for optimal healthy functioning.

Rather than waiting until you feel thirsty, one of the easiest and most accurate ways to know if you need to drink more water is to monitor your urine. If your body has all the water it needs, your urine should be clear and colorless, resembling unsweetened lemonade.

If you are slightly to moderately dehydrated, your urine will generally be yellow. If you are severely, or chronically, dehydrated, your urine will generally appear orange or dark-colored. It is important to note that your urine can change color due to the use of vitamins and other nutritional supplements, often appearing bright yellow when such supplements are used.

Other telltale signs of dehydration are feelings of fatigue, dry skin, and joint and/or muscle aches and pains for no apparent reason, although all of these symptoms can also be signs of other health conditions.

How Much Water Should You Drink?

Based on his findings, Dr. Batmanghelidj advised that all of us should drink at least one-half ounce of water for every pound of our body weight. In addition, he also suggested that people consume a quarter teaspoon of salt per every 32 ounces of water drank per day, to help the body maintain an adequate supply of minerals. (Sea or Celtic salt is best, as these types of salt contain a much wider range of minerals than common table salt does.) The addition of salt increases water absorbability by the cells, thus enhancing water's ability to flush out acidic cellular waste.

As a general rule of thumb, Dr. Batmanghelidj recommended starting each day with two glasses of water and to drink water 20 minutes before eating food, although water with meals is permissible whenever one feels thirsty.

Here are some other guidelines you can follow to keep your body properly hydrated:

- Avoid drinking soda. In addition to being unhealthy for you, soda is also highly dehydrating. The same goes for commercial, non-herbal teas.

- Drink pure, filtered water and avoid water in plastic bottles, as plastic contains unhealthy chemicals that can leech into water.

- Get in the habit of drinking a glass of water 20 to 30 minutes before each meal and another glass 30 to 45 minutes after eating. Doing so supports digestion and also reduces hunger pangs, leading to healthier eating habits. Adding ACV to water before meals will further enhance digestion.

- Limit your consumption of coffee and alcohol, as both beverages are also dehydrating.

- Start your mornings by drinking a large glass of water before breakfast. For an added benefit, add between one teaspoon to one tablespoon of apple cider vinegar.

- Take regular water-drinking breaks throughout the day, especially after each time that you urinate.

REGULAR EXERCISE

Regular and appropriate exercise is essential for good health, and for preventing and reversing most of the health problems afflicting our nation today. The human body is designed for daily physical activity. However, as a nation, we have become increasingly sedentary, which is one of the primary reasons we now face such a daunting health crisis in this country. This alarming trend is especially true of our children, 25 percent of whom are unhealthily, overweight, or obese.

Numerous studies show that sedentary people, on average, don't live as long or enjoy as good health as people who exercise regularly. Based on these studies, a growing number of researchers and physicians now believe that lack of exercise is a more significant risk factor for decreased life expectancy than the *combined risks* of cigarette smoking, high cholesterol, being overweight, and high blood pressure. The scientific evidence conclusively makes one fact very clear: *Being unfit means being unhealthy.*

Here is a breakdown of the many benefits that regular exercise and physical activity can provide:

- Better quality of sleep

- Decreased "fight or flight" response, and therefore less stress

- Improved mental function

- Improved recovery from heart disease and reduced risk of repeat heart conditions

- Improved self-esteem and greater confidence

- Improved balance, especially among older people, and diminishes the risk of falls and injury

- Increased aerobic capacity

- Increased flexibility

- Increased incidence of positive attitudes and emotions, including joy

- Increased longevity

- Increased muscle to fat ratio, making dieting and weight loss easier

- Increased muscular strength

- Increased stamina and energy

- Prevention of and relief from anxiety and depression

- Prevention of and relief from tension

- Prevention of heart disease, cancer, and other serious, degenerative diseases

- Reduced risk of alcoholism and drug addiction

Regular exercise also aids digestion, increases circulation, stimulates the lymphatic system (your body's filtration and purification system), and promotes enhanced levels of positive emotions and balanced mood. Regular exercise of an aerobic nature has been shown to increase serotonin levels in the brain. Serotonin levels are associated with feelings of calm and well-being, improved brain function, and enhanced sleep. Given all of the above benefits, you can see why I strongly recommend that you make regular exercise a priority in your life.

There are three elements that a healthy exercise program needs to address: *muscle strength, aerobic capacity,* and *flexibility.* A healthy exercise routine incorporates a blend of strength training, aerobic, and stretching exercises that work in conjunction with each other to provide you with everything you need to make exercising a primary self-care health tool in your life.

Strength Training

Building and maintaining muscle strength is an essential component of your overall exercise program. This is particularly true as you age. Research shows that strength training helps to maintain healthy hormone levels, improve metabolism, reduce the risk of bone loss, and improves your body's ability to efficiently burn calories.

Weight training (weight lifting and training on weight machines) is perhaps the most popular form of strength training, but you can get many of the same strength-building benefits without the use of such equipment. Moreover, not having to rely on weights and weight machines makes it far likelier that you will commit to your training routine. Healthy strength training exercises that do not require any gym equipment include push-up, chin-ups, stomach crunches, and so forth.

Aerobic Exercise

The word *aerobic* means *with oxygen.* Aerobic exercise refers to prolonged exercise that requires extra oxygen to supply energy to the muscles. In general, aerobic exercise causes moderate shortness of breath, perspiration, and an increase in resting pulse rate.

The primary beneficiary of aerobic exercise is the heart muscle, due to the increased oxygen that such exercise provides to it, as well as the rest of your body. Jogging, bicycling, running on treadmills, and using stair climbers are all popular forms of aerobic exercise, as are swimming and sports, such as tennis, racquetball, and basketball. However, the easiest form of aerobic exercise is walking.

Until recently, it was thought that one had to walk an average of 60 minutes per day to get adequate aerobic benefits. Newer research, however, indicates that you can receive all of the benefits of a 60-minute brisk walk in as little as 15 minutes a day by varying the intensity of your pace. Start by walking at a leisurely pace for about three minutes. Then, for the next minute, walk as fast as you can. Then once more slow down to a leisurely pace for another minute. Continue to alternate between one minute fast and leisurely walking intervals for a total cycle of six times.

Stretching

The final component of your exercise routine involves stretching, which helps to increase and maintain your body's flexibility. This is important because lack of flexibility can severely inhibit your physical performance, lead to poor posture, and increase your risk of injury. In addition, increased flexibility also leads to improved strength and function, allowing your body's muscle groups to operate at peak efficiency. Other benefits of flexibility include improved circulation and greater suppleness of your body's tendons, ligaments, and connective tissues.

There are a variety of exercises that improve flexibility, such as yoga, Tai chi, and various types of bodywork, all of which are excellent. There are also a variety of simple stretching exercises you can do to improve and maintain your body's flexibility on your own. By combining exercises that provide all of the above benefits, you will soon find yourself feeling healthier and more fit than you might believe is possible right now.

Here are some further guidelines you can follow to get the best results from your exercise program. By following these guidelines, you can not only be assured of the best results, but can also be sure of being able to perform your exercise regimen without fear of injury or over-exertion.

If you have an **existing medical condition**, or are just starting to exercise, be sure to consult with your physician prior to beginning the program. Once your doctor has cleared you for exercise, be sure to abide by the following guidelines.

- Adopt a positive attitude about exercise and make it fun. By focusing on the important health benefits that exercise provides, you will enable yourself to more easily achieve them. A positive mindset can also make exercise fun and more enjoyable. You are more likely to continue exercising if you are doing something that you like.

- Avoid exercising, especially aerobic exercises, during times of emotional crises or when you are angry. Exercise under such conditions is counter-productive and can put a dangerous strain on your heart.

- Be sure to start off any work-out/exercise session with proper warm-up and stretching exercises. This will help to avoid post-exercise soreness or injury.

- Breathe! When performing any type of exercise, be sure to breathe in a relaxed, deep manner. Doing so will add to the benefits of the exercise itself by increasing the amount of oxygen that is available for your body's cells, tissues, and organs.

- If you exercise outdoors, be sure to dress appropriately for the weather.

- Just as warming-up and stretching is important as you begin each exercise session, so is a cool-down period at the end of your exercise activity. This should include at least several minutes of gentle stretching or walking.

- Listen to music you enjoy. Listening to such music when your exercise can not only increase your enjoyment during your exercise routine but can also provide you with a soundtrack to enhance your pace and overall performance.

- Wait at least 2 hours after eating before exercising. Additionally, when exercising before meals, wait at least 30 minutes after your exercise session ends before eating. Also drink plenty of water at least half an hour before you begin. You can drink water during the exercise session, if you are thirsty, but do so sparingly.

- Wear the proper attire when exercising, including shoes with the proper support for the activity. Tight clothing and shoes can restrict your circulation and dissipation of heat during exercise. Avoid them.

- When exercising indoors, make sure your room is well ventilated. Open windows or turn on the fan or the air-conditioner during summer months to avoid exercising in a room that is too hot.

By following the above guidelines, you will be sure to get the most benefit from the exercises you perform. Remember, the key to long-term success is to find exercise activities you enjoy and commit to them on a regular basis. As you begin your exercise program, remember that it is important to not try to accomplish too much too soon. Slow and easy is the rule, not "No pain, no gain." As you begin your exercise program stay at your level for at least 5 to 7 days before you increase your activity. This allows you to progress in a safe and effective manner without overtaxing your body.

As I have already mentioned, if you haven't exercised in a long time, be sure to get the advice of your physician first. You may also want to initially train with a fitness coach or other professional. Or you may find exercise becomes more enjoyable if you do it with a friend or family member. Over a period of weeks, as you make exercise a regular part of your daily life, you will find that you can achieve more and will begin to notice improved energy and endurance, as well as increased happiness and personal satisfaction.

ADEQUATE SLEEP

A good night's sleep is one of the most important factors for achieving and maintaining optimal health. It's also often overlooked and, for tens of millions of Americans, very difficult to come by. Here are just some of the reasons why sleep is important for overall health.

- Sleep helps to repair your body.

- Sleep helps keep your heart healthy.

- Sleep reduces stress.

- Sleep improves immune function.

- Sleep improves memory.

- Sleep helps to maintain healthy weight.

Prior to the invention of the light bulb and electric lighting in homes, most Americans averaged 9 hours of sleep each night. Today, especially during the work week, that number has been reduced to 6 or 7 hours of sleep for most Americans, and in some cases much less, especially among people who are middle-aged or older. Yet sleep researchers have found that, with few exceptions, most people require at least 7 to 8 hours of sleep each and every night. That should be your goal, as well.

In order to improve your sleep, it's important that you first understand the factors that may be contributing to poor sleep so that you can address those that may be affecting you. As you read what follows, identify any of the factors that apply to you and apply the relevant action steps that address them.

Diet

Poor diet and/or poor eating habits, such as eating late in the evening, only a few hours before retiring, can often cause or exacerbate sleeping problems. This is especially true of the standard American diet, which is high in salt, sugars, simple and refined carbohydrates, unhealthy oils, convenience, processed foods, and lacking in organic fresh fruits and vegetables.

Excessive alcohol and caffeine intake can also cause sleep problems. Alcohol can disrupt your body's circadian rhythms and interfere with healthy REM sleep, while caffeine is a known stimulant that can leave you feeling on edge and unable to properly relax, thus preventing and interfering with sleep. Caffeine, in particular, has been linked by researchers to insomnia, periodic limb movement in sleep, and restless legs syndrome.

Food Allergies and Sensitivities

Food allergies and sensitivities can interfere with your ability to sleep peacefully and restfully and are a frequent cause of sleep disorders.

Among the ways that food allergies and sensitivities can cause or worsen sleeping problems are the hypoglycemia (low blood sugar) they can cause, as well as increased histamine production. Sugar and carbohydrate foods are frequent triggers of food allergies that cause drops in blood sugar levels. When this happens, the body compensates by producing spikes in insulin production. This creates an adrenal stress reaction that puts the body in a state of stimulation characterized by jittery feelings and tension.

During allergic food reactions, the body can also produce elevated levels of histamine in the brain, disrupting brain chemistry. This, in turn, can greatly affect your ability to get a good night's sleep, and can often result in insomnia.

The most common foods that produce allergies and sensitivities are caffeine, chocolate, corn, dairy products, eggs, wheat, and wheat products, as well as sugars and refined carbohydrates. Any food can potentially trigger such reactions, however. If you suffer from sleep problems that are accompanied by fatigue during the day (especially upon awakening and throughout the morning) and/or frequent feelings of irritability, most likely your condition is being caused or exacerbated by food allergies or sensitivities.

If you suspect that you suffer from food allergies, try eliminating the suspect foods above from your diet. Do this for one month and note any improvements to your sleep, health, and energy levels during that time. If problems persist, consider working with a food allergy specialist or a doctor trained in environmental medicine. You can locate such physicians by contacting the American Academy of Environmental Medicine at www.aaemonline.org.

Lack of Exercise

Lack of regular exercise typically results in chronic muscle tension and the buildup of stress in the body, which can make relaxing and falling asleep more difficult.

Overstimulation Before You Go to Bed

Over-stimulating yourself before you go to bed can make falling asleep more difficult. There are a variety of ways in which you can over-stimulate yourself, including late night exercise, watching television, or working on your computer, including checking your email. All of these activities serve to stimulate brain function by generating "busy mode" beta wave activity. While beta wave activity is essential for problem-solving and dealing with many other issues during waking hours, quick and restful sleep can only occur when beta waves in the brain subside, giving way to the more relaxed states of alpha and theta waves. (A fourth type of brain wave, known as delta wave, occurs during deep, dreamless sleep.)

To prevent overstimulation, get in the habit of spending the last 30 minutes of your day in "quiet time" activities, such as mediation, prayer, or other relaxing activities that you enjoy. Doing so on a regular basis will start to prime both your brain and body to more readily shift towards sleep as you let go of the cares of the day.

Creating An Optimal Sleep Environment

Your bedroom may be an overlooked factor that is contributing to unhealthy sleep. Here are some guidelines you can use to transform your bedroom into a more conducive sleep environment:

■ Keep your bedroom clean and free of dust. This means cleaning your bedroom at least once a week and washing blankets, sheets, and pillow cases frequently as well. An unclean bedroom not only interferes with restful sleep, it also makes you more susceptible to infectious microorganisms and can negatively impact your respiratory system as you breathe in dust while you are sleeping. To further prevent dust build up consider using an air purifier in your home, and also be sure that the filters on your heat ducts are professionally examined at least once a year and replaced as necessary.

■ Be sure to allow for a flow of fresh air throughout your bedroom as you sleep. You can do this easily by keeping at least one window of your bedroom slightly open as you sleep. Breathing fresh, oxygen-rich air when you go to bed will not only enhance the benefits of sleep itself but also make it easier for you to fall asleep.

■ Sleep on a comfortable mattress. What makes a mattress comfortable is a subjective experience. Simply put, you will know what type of mattress is most comfortable for you when you experience it. Despite the investment in a new mattress, if your current mattress is uncomfortable you will find the cost of a new mattress that meets your specific needs well worth it.

■ Be aware that you might be sensitive to the materials in your pillow, blankets, and sheets. As a general rule, cotton or wool blankets and sheets and feather pillows are healthier choices than the same items made from synthetic materials.

■ Make sure that the temperature in your bedroom is kept at a comfortable level. Temperatures that are too hot or cold can significantly interfere with your ability to get a good night's sleep.

- Make your bedroom a place of sleep, not a place to watch television. If you have a TV in your bedroom, consider moving it to another room in your home. Watching TV in bed keeps your brain in active mode, making sleep more difficult to come by once you turn in for the night.

- In addition to removing a TV from your bedroom, if you have one there, also try to keep your bedroom free of other electrical appliances, such as stereos, cell phones, computer, radios. Again, your bedroom should be a place of sleep, not an entertainment or work center. Moreover, a growing body of research indicates that sleeping in a room full of electrical appliances can interfere with healthy, restorative sleep because of the electromagnetic frequencies such devices emit, even when they are not in use.

- These frequencies can cause what is now recognized as electromagnetic pollution that can negatively impact your body on an energetic level, making sleep more difficult, and also devitalizing you by draining your body's own energy. At the very least, be sure to sleep at least eight feet away from all such devices, if you feel you must have them in your bedroom, and also unplug them before you retire for the night. For best results, though, banish all such devices from your bedroom.

- Sleep in the dark. This means not only turning off your bedroom lights when you go to bed, but also making sure that curtains and shades are fully drawn as well to prevent outdoor light from entering your bedroom. Sleeping in complete darkness helps your body to produce the hormone melatonin, which is essential for healthy sleep, as well as many other functions in your body.

Take a look at your bedroom to see how well it meets the above guidelines. Then, if improvements need to be made, please be sure to make them.

Diet and Sleeping-Promoting Foods and Beverages

One of the keys to a restful night's sleep is to calm your brain. Certain foods contribute to restful sleep because they are rich in tryptophan. Tryptophan is an amino acid that the body uses to make serotonin, the neurotransmitter that slows down nerve signals so that your brain is able to relax. Tryptophan is also a precursor of melatonin. Although it is not advisable to have a full meal within a few hours of your bedtime, having a light snack of tryptophan-rich foods is permissible.

Turkey is a food that is rich in tryptophan (which explains why so many people feel ready for a nap soon after they finish their Thanksgiving meal). A small turkey sandwich eaten an hour or more before you go to bed, along with a cup of herbal tea, can be a delicious way to prepare for a good night's sleep.

Other tryptophan-rich foods include chicken, chickpeas, eggs, fish, lentils, milk, and yogurt. Certain nuts and seeds, such as almonds, hazelnuts, pumpkin seeds, sesame seeds, and sunflower seeds also contain tryptophan and can therefore boost serotonin levels and enhance sleep when snacked on before bed. Just be sure not to overdo your snacking.

Another way to improve sleep has been recommended by practitioners of yoga for centuries. Pour a cup of milk into a pan and warm it just before it starts to boil. Then pour the milk into a cup and add a teaspoon of raw honey. Let the mixture cool for a few minutes, and then sip it slowly a few minutes before bedtime. This remedy has a very calming effect. If you are *lactose intolerant,* you can substitute almond milk for regular milk and still get the same benefits.

Any of the above snacks can help ready your brain, and therefore your body, for sleep. Choose whichever ones most appeal you. Also be sure to follow the dietary recommendations shared earlier in this chapter.

Sleep-Enhancing Herbs and Nutrients

Various herbs are also well-known for their ability to promote restful sleep. They include chamomile, hops, lavender, lemon balm, passionflower, skullcap, and valerian root, all of which can be prepared as teas.

A variety of nutrients are also known to improve and restore sleep. Among the best researched nutrients for sleep promotion are B vitamins (especially vitamins B5 and B6), vitamin E, magnesium, and an amino acid known as GABA. Individual B vitamins are best taken with a complete B-complex formula to enhance their benefits. They can be taken at any time during the day or night.

Taking a Bath for Better Sleep

Taking a bath before bedtime can significantly improve the quality of your sleep. This fact was conclusively shown to be true in a survey conducted in 1999 by the National Sleep Foundation. The survey found that respondents who took a hot bath before going to bed overwhelmingly reported that they fell asleep more quickly and easily and slept better than usual.

Other studies have found that taking a hot bath before bedtime can raise core body temperature by approximately 2 degrees F, and that hot baths at night also increase the production of melatonin, the most important hormone necessary for healthy sleep. This increase in melatonin production was found to be caused as a natural reaction of the brain's pineal gland to increased body temperature caused by hot baths. The end result is a state of enhanced relaxation that carries over into better and deeper sleep.

You can add some of the herbs mentioned above to your bath to get even more sleep-enhancing benefits. To do so combine one to two tablespoons of each of the dry, loose herbs and place the mixture in a muslin bag. Tie the bag closed and then place it in your bathtub as it fills with hot water. Keep the bag in the tub as you soak in it for 20 minutes. Not only will this herbal bath promote relaxation, it will also help to ease any muscle tension you may have. For even better results, have a cup of chamomile tea while you are soaking.

Here is an alternative method you can also try. Instead of using herbs, pour two cups of Epsom salts into your bath as it fills with hot water. Then soak in the solution for 20 minutes. Epsom salts contain a high amount of magnesium, a mineral that has potent relaxant properties. As you soak in the hot water, the magnesium contained in the salts will be absorbed into your body through your skin.

I cannot overemphasize how vitally important adequate levels of deep, restful sleep is to your overall health. In many ways, it may very well be the most vital component of healthy lifestyle, perhaps even more so than a healthy diet, because without quality sleep your body's numerous health functions, including digesting the foods you eat and assimilating their nutrients, simply cannot occur at optimum levels due to the stressors that chronic poor sleep cause.

By following the above guidelines, you should hopefully find the quality of your sleep improving within a few weeks to a month. If, after that time, you continue to experience sleep problems, I strongly advise that you speak with your doctor.

STRESS MANAGEMENT

According to the Centers for Disease Control and Prevention (CDC), stress is the primary cause of 85 percent of all diseases, and 90 percent of all visits to primary care physicians in the U.S. are directly due to stress-related complaints. In addition, according to a landmark 20-year study conducted by researchers at the University of London, unmanaged stress is a more serious risk factor for both heart disease and cancer than either cigarette smoking or frequent consumption of high cholesterol foods.

However, despite the compelling scientific evidence linking stress to illness, little attention to managing stress is usually given by doctors when they consult with their patients. Although doctors may counsel their patients to try to relax more, rarely do they provide them with effective self-care tools for doing so. Instead, they may prescribe tranquilizing drugs, which can provide temporary relief, but do not address the underlying problem. Fortunately, there is much that you can do on your own to better manage stress.

Mental and Emotional Stress

In the vast majority of cases, it is not physical stress that is at the heart of disease, but mental and emotional stress. To better understand how thoughts and beliefs can influence your health for good or bad, let's take a closer look at how the body is designed to protect itself from disease, starting with your body's immune system. Your immune system is your human body's first line of defense against disease. Its task is to identify invading microorganisms (bacteria, fungi, parasites, and viruses) and to attack and eliminate them before they can cause harm to the body's cells, tissues, and organs.

"Flight or Fight" Response

Important as the immune system is to good health, however, there is another body system that is equally as, and perhaps even more, important. This system is known as the hypothalamus-pituitary-adrenal (HPA) axis. The purpose of the HPA axis is to spring into action at the first sign of any external threats that the body may face. When there aren't any threats, the HPA axis is in what might be described as "idle mode." This state of idleness allows the rest of your body to flourish the way that nature intended. But when the hypothalamus center in the brain perceives an outside threat, it signals the HPA axis to "roll out" and do its job. This is known as the "flight or fight" response.

As soon as this signal is given, your body's adrenal glands increase their production of cortisol and other stress hormones, releasing them into the blood stream. Once this happens, blood vessels that supply oxygen and nutrients to your body's cells and organs are constricted so that more blood can be made available to nourish the tissues of your body's arms and legs, since it is primarily these extremities that the body uses to fend off external attacks and get out of harm's way.

Prior to this response, the blood in the body is concentrated in what are known as the visceral organs. These are the organs responsible for digestion and absorption of foods and nutrients, excretion, and various other functions that provide for proper cell growth and production of cellular energy. As blood is rushed to the tissues of the arms and legs, the visceral organs, such as the stomach, kidneys, and liver, cannot function at 100 percent, causing all growth-related activities in the body to become limited.

As you can imagine, if this process continues for sustained periods of time, your body's overall functioning will start to suffer. But this situation is further compounded by the impact sustained "flight or fight" responses have on the immune system. During "flight or fight" responses, the HPA axis causes the adrenal glands to suppress immune function in order to conserve the body's energy reserves via the adrenals increased production of stress hormones.

While the "flight or fight" response played an essential role in helping to keep our ancestors alive in the face of physical dangers, today most of us are not faced with such dangers, and even when we are, they are usually short-lived events. However, researchers have discovered that actual physical danger is not necessary to trigger the "flight or fight" response. It can also be triggered by your thoughts and beliefs. Simply put, if you habitually focus on thoughts and beliefs of a limiting or negative nature, you are causing your body to act as if it is in danger.

Chronically elevated stress hormones results in a chronically suppressed immune function, leading to a greater susceptibility to infectious disease. Additionally, because of how the organs of the body are also negatively impacted by chronic stress, many other functions are also suppressed, setting the stage for impaired digestion, increased muscle tension, and eventual declines in cell and tissue function, which can lead to a wide range of diseases, including heart attack and cancer.

Dealing With Stress

Based on these facts it's clear that one of the most important steps you can take to ensure your health is to deal with stress effectively. To do so, you first must become better aware of the types of stress to which you are most commonly exposed. The most common types of stress are:

- **Emotional stress**, which includes suppressed or inappropriately expressed emotions, such as anger, anxiety, depression, fear, and guilt; divorce or other breakups; death; suffering on the part of those you care for; chronic illness (yours or some you love); lack of nurturing relationships/friends; and unresolved life issues from the past.

- **Environmental stress**, such as exposure to allergens, chemicals and other environmental toxins, as well as fluorescent lights, computer and computer printers, cell phones, and other household appliances.

- **Physical stress**, which includes allergens, temperature (too hot or too cold), physical inactivity, illness, physical pain or trauma, and lack of sleep.

- **Social stress**, such as relationship issues with a spouse or significant other, family members and friends; issues with co-workers; unpleasant neighbors; job promotions or demotions; financial issues; and politics.

- **Spiritual stress**, such as not knowing your life's purpose, fear of death and/or the afterlife, lack of faith, and a variety of other existential issues, all of which can cause or worsen a spiritual crisis.

When it comes to stress, it's often not the events that occur in your life that cause stress, but how you *react* to those events. Many times, the events, by themselves, are neutral. It's how you think about them that determines whether or not they will cause stress in your life. By changing your attitude related to your thoughts, you can reduce or eliminate stress.

Thinking Patterns

Thoughts that cause stress are usually a form of what psychologists refer to as *distorted thinking.* This means seeing things not as they are, but as we *choose to think they are.* By recognizing the role that your thoughts play in determining your reactions to what you experience in your life, you can understand why learning to consciously choose your thoughts can make a big difference in the degree to which stress affects you. The most common distorted thinking patterns are:

Blameful thinking. People who think from a blameful perspective hold themselves or others responsible for every problem that comes their way, even when neither they nor others are to blame. Usually, blame also prevents them from moving on from past situations, and can also result in an inability to take responsibility for their present experiences.

Emotional reasoning. This distorted thinking pattern is characterized by a belief that whatever you feel must be true. While feelings certainly can be valuable clues to what is true in our lives, automatically accepting your feelings as true is not always advisable.

Negative thinking. Negative thinking involves focusing on the negative details related to the events and people we encounter, to the point where all positive details are filtered out. This leads to a distorted magnification of the negative details, making them worse than they actually are. People who are negative thinkers tend to willfully refuse to see "the bright side" of people or events. Such thinking can create and perpetuate stress.

Personalization. This type of distorted thinking is characterized by the belief that everything people do or say is some kind of reaction to you. People who think in this manner take everything personally, perceiving slights, insults, and other negative intentions from people even when that is not the case at all.

Polarized thinking. This type of distorted thinking is characterized by seeing things in "absolutes." People whose thinking is polarized tend to see things as "black or white," "good or bad," "sinful or spiritual," and so forth. When polarized thinking is present, there are no "grey areas" and no middle ground. Polarized thinkers are usually unable to view anything and anyone without automatically deciding that events and people are "good" or "bad" and therefore stressful or not stressful, *regardless of objective reality.* Unfair as this can be to those people polarized thinkers determine are "bad," it is often even worse for the polarized thinkers themselves.

"Should have" thinking. People who think from a "should have" perspective tend to have a list of ironclad rules about how they and other people should act. People who break these rules anger them. Additionally, they feel guilty if they violate the rules themselves.

Victim thinking. This type of thinking is common in people who view themselves as helpless when it comes to certain people or events. People who think in this way believe they have no control over what happens to them, when in fact they do. Victim thinking prevents them from recognizing their ability to take control of their lives.

All of the above types of distorted thinking create "lose-lose" situations that can turn neutral, and even positive, situations and social interactions into stressful ones.

Once you have identified the distorted thinking patterns that you are prone to, ask yourself what patterns of distorted thinking might be involved in the stressors that are most common in your life. Then ask yourself if the stressors would have the same effects on you if the way you think about them wasn't distorted. Take your time with this exercise and be honest with yourself as you go through it. If you are, you might be surprised to discover that at least some of your stressors on your list needn't be stressful at all.

Reframing

A powerful method you can use to free yourself from distorted thinking is known as reframing. Simply put, reframing is a process that will help you to see things in a different way than you have seen them in the past. More specifically, reframing helps to remove the judgments that are the principal causes of distorted thinking patterns. You can use reframing with any situation that throws you out of balance and causes stress, whether it's a relationship issue, work-related, or an unexpected event.

There are three steps in reframing process you can use to eliminate or defuse distorted thinking patterns.

1. The first step is to simply recognize and admit to distorted thinking when you find yourself doing it. Then, instead of just automatically reacting to the situation that triggered it, no matter how charged or tense or uncomfortable you feel because of the situation, take a moment to notice how your thoughts are contributing to what you are feeling. Next, recognize that you have a choice in how you are responding to the situation at hand. You can also take a few deep breaths to help yourself calm down and relax. This will prepare you for step two.

2. As you contemplate the situation that is triggering your stress, take time to consider all the possible ways you can deal with it. Remember, you are not a victim of circumstance and you always have a choice in how you respond to whatever life brings you. Knowing that, look at each potential response that you come up with and ask yourself, "Which is most appropriate for me? Which one will get me closer to my goal? Which one best serves me and brings me peace of mind?" Then choose accordingly.

3. The third step is practice. Distorted thinking habits do not occur overnight. Usually they are ingrained, unconscious patterns that have been with us for most of our lives. Therefore, it is unrealistic to assume you can get rid of them without a bit of time and effort. This is why practice is so important. The more you practice consciously examining your thought patterns, the more you will develop the ability to choose how you want to think about—and therefore respond to—people and situations that in the past triggered stressful reactions within you. Awareness is the key.

Lifestyle Tips

What follow are other simple, yet highly effective, lifestyle tips you can use to both reduce stress in your life and manage it better. By incorporating the following guidelines into your daily routine you will soon begin to feel and be more stress-free.

- Avoid long periods of isolation, especially if you live alone. Seek out and enjoy your friends and loved ones.

- Be sure to get enough sleep and try to go to bed at the same time each night.

- Cultivate laughter in your daily life and make a conscious effort to find the humor in things.

- Don't be afraid of compromising, especially about matters that aren't significant.

- Don't be afraid to discuss your situation with your family or friends, or to ask for help if you need it.

- Don't skip breakfast and be sure the foods you eat are healthy for you.

- Exercise for at least 30 minutes for a minimum of three days each week.

- Find a hobby you enjoy and commit to pursuing it on a regular basis.

- Identify your fears and worries and examine them objectively. In most cases, you will find doing so will make them far less significant and much more manageable.

- Know what's most essential and important in your life and commit yourself to that instead of wasting time on matters that are unimportant.

- Make a commitment to yourself and those you care about to be more loving.

- Once you decide to do something, act on it as soon as possible. Hesitations about taking action can dramatically ramp up your stress levels.

- Regularly engage in relaxation exercises and/or meditation.

- Schedule your day so that you have free time to relax and spend with your loved ones.

- Set up your daily schedule so that you have plenty of time to devote to your daily tasks, instead of having to hurry to meet your responsibilities.

Be assertive in the requests you make so that you are treated with respect and taken seriously by others. And keep in mind that everybody is stressed to some degree. Recognizing this fact makes it easier to realize that the stress you may be experiencing is far from unique. By sharing your issues with others you will likely discover answers to your problems from those who have also faced them. In turn, you may also be able to provide them with your own helpful insights.

Physical exercise is another excellent means of reducing stress, so long as you do not overdo it. One of the easiest and most effective exercises you can use to release stress is to go for a walk. Besides being one of the most effective ways to exercise, walking can also be very relaxing. In addition, many people who regularly take walks find that it helps them to come up with new solutions to their challenges and problems.

Other ways that you can more effectively manage stress include meditation exercises, deep breathing exercises, laughter and developing a sense of humor, keeping a diary or journal, listening to music, taking a nap, getting a massage, spending time with family members and friends whose company you enjoy, and, of course, getting enough sleep and eating a healthy diet.

By making a commitment to incorporating at least some of the above stress-busting you will soon find yourself more easily dealing with stress whenever it arises, and also more resistant to stress in the first place. In turn, as your stress levels diminish, your levels of health will increase, as will positive feelings of contentment, joy, and accomplishment.

WORKING WITH YOUR DOCTOR

While all of the above guidelines and recommendations can be used by you to create an overall healthy lifestyle on your own, I also recommend that you work with your doctor to monitor your health status. At a minimum, it is a good idea to schedule a complete annual physical so that you and your doctor can properly assess your overall health status and screen for early signs of disease.

Ideally, your physician will be trained to screen for and treat nutritional imbalances, something that most conventionally trained physicians have little to no experience in. Nor do most dieticians. I recommend seeking out a doctor who makes nutritional assessment an essential component of his or her screening program, and who is also well qualified to determine the diet and nutritional treatment program that is best suited for your unique needs. Remember, during the entire course of conventional medical skill, conventional physicians receive an average of only 25 hours of education in diet and nutrition, which is hardly adequate to meet the needs of their patients. So be sure to ask your doctor about his or her training in this area and, if you aren't satisfied, seek out another doctor. Your best bet is to work with a physician with a background in either integrative or functional medicine. Naturopathic physicians and clinical nutritionists can also be very helpful to work with. Many chiropractors are also trained in nutritional medicine. Ideally, your physician should also be skilled in screening for and treating hormone imbalances.

Recommended for Women

When taking your annual physical, it is recommended that your blood tests include the following:

- CBC (complete blood count) test
- Chem profile

- Insulin testing
- DHEA-S
- 25 OH Vitamin D
- Cortisol
- HGB A1C
- Hs CRP (C-reactive protein)
- HDL, LDL, Total Cholesterol
- Homocysteine
- Mg RBC (magnesium red blood cell test)*
- Triglycerides
- IgF1, IGFPB3

- Free T3, TSH
- Thyroid Peroxidase
- Thyroglobulin Antibody
- Estradiol
- Progesterone
- FSH (follicle stimulating hormone)
- LH (luteinizing hormone)
- SHBG (sex hormone binding globulin)
- Prolactin
- Testosterone/Free Testosterone

* This is not the same as a serum magnesium test, and is a far better indicator of your body's magnesium status; magnesium is one of the most important nutrients for your body, being essential for over 300 vital functions.

The best time to draw blood for testing in women who are still menstruating is on day 20 or 21 of your menstrual cycle.

Recommended for Men

For men, all of the above tests are recommended, with the exception of progesterone and FSH. Men should also receive the PSA and Free PSA blood tests.

By working proactively with your doctor and partaking of an annual comprehensive physical you will go a long way to better ensuring that you live a long and healthy life.

CONCLUSION

Now let's turn our attention back to apple cider vinegar and its many benefits as a treatment for a wide variety of health conditions and other uses. That is the focus in the next section, Part Two, where you will learn how you can use apple cider vinegar to relieve the symptoms of more than 80 health disorders.

A-to-Z Guide
of Health Conditions

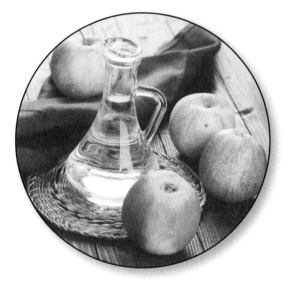

In this section you will learn how apple cider vinegar can help relieve more than 80 health conditions. In each of the conditions that follow, I will also share with you potential factors you may need to consider in order to get the complete relief you are looking for. Remember, apple cider vinegar is not a cure-all, yet it *can* often be highly effective for dealing with these conditions. However, if your condition persists, please consult your doctor for more assistance.

ACID REFLUX

Acid reflux, more commonly known as heartburn, is a condition that most people experience at least once in their lives. However, especially because of the poor eating habits of many Americans today, acid reflux is becoming increasingly common and many people experience it on a frequent, recurring basis. Severe, recurrent flare-ups of acid reflux can lead to gastro-esophageal reflux disease (GERD), a serious health condition that, if left untreated, can cause esophageal (throat) cancer, a type of cancer that used to be relatively rare, but which has increased in occurrence by more than 600 percent in the U.S. over the past 30 years.

Symptoms

In most cases, it causes fleeting sensations of discomfort and usually resolves on its own, typically within 20 minutes to 1 to 2 hours. You may experience:

- Abdominal pain in the upper region
- Acid indigestion or heartburn
- Acid backing up in your throat or regurgitation
- Bloating or stomach fullness
- Burping
- Nausea after consuming food

Causes

Acid reflux is caused by stomach acid moving back up into the esophagus, instead of staying in the stomach where it belongs. Each time you swallow while eating or drinking, a circular muscle valve located around the bottom part of the esophagus relaxes, allowing food and liquids to pass into your stomach. Under normal conditions, once food or drink has entered your stomach, this valve, which is known as the lower esophageal sphincter, or LES, then closes to prevent stomach acid (primarily hydrochloric acid) from backing up into your throat. Acid reflux occurs when the LES does not close properly, resulting in a burning sensation in the throat that can sometimes also be felt in the chest. GERD occurs when the LES frequently does not close properly. Over time, GERD can thin the lining of the esophagus, which, in turn, can result in throat cancer if not treated in time.

Benefits

Given that both acid reflux and GERD are caused by stomach acid backing up into the throat, it may seem odd that apple cider vinegar, which is also acidic by nature, can help relieve acid reflux and, in some cases, even GERD. Yet, as many people have reported, very often, it can.

Although to my knowledge no research has been conducted on ACV as a treatment for acid reflux, there is an extensive body of anecdotal evidence from patient testimonials claiming that apple cider vinegar can relieve symptoms of acid reflux and GERD. There are two possible reasons that may explain how and why ACV provides such relief. One theory is that the acetic acid in apple cider vinegar lowers stomach acidity since acetic acid is a weaker acid than hydrochloric acid. This makes sense, given that acetic acid along with its acetate salt can help buffer and maintain stomach acid at a pH level of about 3.0. At this pH range the stomach still has enough acid to digest food but not enough to trigger acid reflux.

Conversely, another possible explanation lies in the theory that the LES is pH sensitive, and that when the stomach lacks enough acid to properly digest food, the LES valve does not receive the signals from the acid that cause it to close properly after swallowing. This also makes sense, since it is typically older age groups that more commonly experience acid reflux and GERD. As we age, the amount of hydrochloric acid produced by our stomachs usually declines. Apple cider vinegar can supply added acid, thus providing the LES valve with the acidity signaling it needs to function properly.

Whatever the reason, if you suffer from acid reflux or GERD, the only way to know whether or not ACV can help you is to try it and see for yourself.

ACV Treatment

Add between one teaspoon to one or two tablespoons of ACV (start with the lower dose and increase if needed) to one eight-ounce glass of pure, filtered water, and drink it 20 minutes before each meal. Try to do this before every meal. If ACV is going to work with you, doing this should help prevent reflux flare-ups or minimize their severity within a few days to a few weeks. If you do experience reflux after you eat, you can also try drinking ACV in water when symptoms occur.

What Else to Consider

Persistent or frequently recurring reflux can be a sign of a more serious underlying condition, such as hiatal hernia, food allergies and sensitivities, poor digestion, impaired liver function, and stomach and other gastrointestinal infections. Being overweight or obese can also cause reflux, as can smoking, and eating overly large meals, as well as excessive protein intake, spicy foods, and foods rich in unhealthy fats.

ACNE

Long the bane of self-conscious teenagers, acne is a skin condition caused by bacterial buildup and inflammation within the skin's sebaceous glands, which are located deep within the pores of the skin. Sebaceous glands produce sebum, an oil that keeps skin soft and moist. As with all of the other organs of your body, your skin, which is your body's largest organ, is constantly renewing itself, with old skin cells dying and shed off to be replaced by new skin cells. Under normal circumstances this process is gradual and occurs evenly. Sometimes, though, skin sheds unevenly, causing dead skin cells to mix with sebum, trapping oil and bacteria inside skin pores. The end result is acne. All told, approximately 90 percent of all teenagers, and 25 percent of adults in America will experience acne at some point.

Symptoms

Acne can occur anywhere on the body, but most commonly is found on the face and neck in the form of red or whitish pimples and blackheads. The signs differ, determined by the severity of the skin problem, and the following may appear:

- Blackheads
- Pimples
- Pus-filled lumps beneath the skin that may cause pain (cystic lesions)

- Red bumps
- Solid large bumps beneath the skin (nodules)

Causes

Because of changes in hormone levels, especially during puberty, hormones can accelerate the activity of oil-producing sebaceous glands which is why teenagers have a particularly high risk for acne. Although the teenage years are when outbreaks of acne are most likely to occur, acne can strike at any time, especially in people who eat an unhealthy diet and/or who are nutritionally deficient. Acne can also occur, both prior to and before the onset of a woman's monthly menstrual cycle and during times of excessive stress. It is one of the most common health conditions in the U.S. today, as evidenced by the fact that the total cost of acne treatments in the United States per year is estimated to be $1.4 billion, with over $100 million of that sum being spent on over-the-counter acne products. Fortunately, in many cases, apple cider vinegar can offer an effective and very inexpensive alternative.

Benefits

Apple cider vinegar, applied topically, acts as a natural skin toner and can help prevent and banish acne flare-ups in four interrelated ways.

- First, it acts as a natural *astringent* and is effective for removing dead skin cells.

- Second, it helps to balance skin pH so that your skin does not become too acidic or alkaline. In fact, the pH of ACV is close to the natural pH of skin, so when ACV is applied to skin it helps to maintain what is called the skin's acid mantle, which protects against foreign bacteria.

- Third, it helps cleanse skin pores and removes oils that may be clogging them.

- Finally, ACV helps to reduce inflammation associated with skin blemishes while simultaneously improve circulation in the skin, further helping to reduce acne blemishes.

ACV provides these benefits due to its combination of acids, nutrients, and enzymes it contains. These same ingredients are also supplied when ACV is consumed as a tonic in water.

ACV Treatment

To make a topical ACV *solution,* combine one part ACV with one part water (for example, a quarter cup of ACV with a quarter cup of water). Then dip a clean cotton ball in the solution and gently daub the mixture on the acne blemishes. Allow the mixture to dry on its own. Repeat each morning and evening. This same solution can be used as a natural skin cleanser and toner. (For some people with sensitive skin, the one to one ratio of ACV to water may be too strong. Therefore, initially apply the solution on a small area of your skin as a test solution. If it proves to be too strong, you can further dilute the ACV by increasing the amount of water in the solution.)

For acne on other areas of the body an ACV *bath soak* can also be helpful. Simply add three to four cups of ACV to warm bath water, then soak in it for 20 to 30 minutes.

Drinking one or more glasses of ACV *tonic* (between one teaspoon to two tablespoons of ACV, depending on your tolerance, added to eight ounces of pure, filtered water) each day can provide further benefit.

What Else to Consider

Persistent acne and other skin blemishes can be caused by poor diet, food allergies and sensitivities, nutritional deficiencies, chronic stress, and/or hormone imbalances. Various cosmetic products can also trigger acne flare-ups due to the synthetic ingredients they contain.

AGE SPOTS

Age spots, as their name suggests, are a common occurrence as we age, especially after age 40, but younger people can get them also, as a result of increased exposure to the sun. They typically appear as small, brown splotches on the skin, usually on the face.

Symptoms

Generally age spots occur in people with fair skin, but can also appear in those with a darker complexion. They typically appear on the back of hands, tops of feet, on shoulders, upper back, and face. They appear as flat, oval areas commonly tan or brown. They range from the size of a freckle to a more prominent size.

Benefits

Topical ACV solutions can help reduce age spots for the same reason that topical ACV can work as a treatment for acne. The topical treatment is the same as for acne above.

ACV Treatment

Create an ACV *solution* of one part ACV with one part water, then, using a clean cotton ball, daub the age spots with the solution and allow it to dry on its own. For best results, apply the solution two to three times each day. For most people, the results will not be immediate, so you need to be persistent. After a few weeks, however, you should note some degree of improvement. For further benefit, consume a glass of ACV in water one or more times a day.

What Else to Consider

Age spots can be caused by too much exposure to sunlight, so if you are in the sun a lot, consider wearing a hat to minimize sunlight exposure on your face. Age spots can also be a sign of organ toxicity and/or sluggish liver function.

ALLERGIES

Allergies have become increasingly common in the United States over the last few decades. Today, according to the American Academy of Allergy, Asthma, and Immunology, over 20 percent of children and adults in the U.S. suffer from some type of allergy. Simply put, an allergy is a negative reaction in the body's immune system to one or more substances that under normal circumstances are harmless, including foods and beverages.

Symptoms

Allergy symptoms can be quite varied, ranging from coughing, sneezing, watery eyes, congestion, stuffy nose and swollen sinuses, to itching, fatigue, and rashes. Chronic allergic reactions can also trigger or exacerbate a wide range of other disease conditions, ranging from asthma and other respiratory conditions to arthritis, headache, migraine, weight gain, depression, and many other conditions.

Causes

Allergies should not be taken lightly, and in most cases can only be fully resolved with the help of a trained allergy specialist who will work with you to determine your specific allergy triggers and how best to neutralize them. A wide range of potential factors (allergens) can be involved, such as:

- Animal dander
- Common household products containing chemicals
- Beauty products
- Dust mite casings
- Environmental toxins
- Foods and beverages
- Mold
- Pharmaceutical drugs (especially antibiotics and non-steroidal anti-inflammatory drugs, also known as NSAIDs)
- Pollen
- Tobacco smoke

Benefits

By no means should apple cider vinegar be regarded as a cure for allergies. However, many allergy sufferers report a lessening of their allergy symptoms after drinking an ACV tonic. This is most likely due to ACV's antibacterial and antiviral properties, as well as its ability to improve the body's acid alkaline balance. Additionally, the acetic acid in ACV can also help reduce mucus buildup. Mucus production is a common factor during an allergy attack. ACV's ability to thin mucus is very similar to the mechanism of action of common antihistamine drugs that are often used in the treatment of allergies, meaning that ACV acts as a natural antihistamine.

ACV Treatment

To determine if ACV *tonic* will help relieve your allergy symptoms, combine one tablespoon of ACV with eight ounces of pure filtered water, and drink three times a day, beginning in the morning before breakfast. For added benefit, you might try adding a tablespoon of raw, organic honey to the mixture, since honey also acts as natural immune system booster. (Heat the water first so that the honey dissolves, then add the ACV once the water cools and stir everything together.)

What Else to Consider

Allergies are usually caused by multiple factors in combination with a weakened immune system. Therefore, if you suffer from allergies, it is vitally important that you consult with an allergy specialist to ensure the most effective and comprehensive treatment.

ARTHRITIS

Arthritis is a painful inflammation and stiffness of the joints. It is a term given to more than 100 types of arthritic conditions, with the three most common classes of arthritis being osteoarthritis (the most prevalent form), rheumatoid arthritis, and gout.

Symptoms

Signs or symptoms depend upon the type of arthritis.

Common symptoms of *osteoarthritis* may include joint pain and a gradual development of stiffness.

Rheumatoid arthritis is characterized by inflammation and painful swelling and stiffness in extremities.

The most common signs of *gout* are swelling, tenderness, warmth, and redness in a joint, usually in the big toe.

Causes

Arthritis is a serious, chronic, degenerative disease, and can be caused by a variety of factors, ranging from environmental toxins, poor diet, food allergies and sensitivities, infections, hormone imbalances, and injury.

Osteoarthritis is characterized by a breakdown of cartilage, the smooth, gelatin-like tissue that prevents bones from rubbing against each other.

Rheumatoid arthritis is an autoimmune disease that is caused when the body's immune system attacks its own healthy tissues. It most commonly

affects ligaments and tendons and joints composed of connective tissue, causing them to become inflamed and, in some cases, deformed.

Gout is a form of arthritis that is caused by the buildup of uric acids in
the body. Eventually, this buildup can result in the uric acid becoming crys-
tallized in joint cartilage and fluid, causing sharp, stabbing pains in the joints.

Benefits

While apple cider vinegar is certainly no cure for arthritis, is can sometimes
alleviate arthritis symptoms, particularly those related to osteoarthritis and
gout. When ACV works in this regard, it most likely does so by neutralizing
the buildup of acids in the body due to its alkalizing effect once it is consumed
and metabolized. This, in turn, can help break down uric acid crystals and
alleviate symptoms of inflammation.

ACV Treatment

To relieve arthritis symptoms, combine one to two tablespoons of ACV with
eight ounces of pure, filtered water, and drink two to three glasses each day.
If you suffer from gout, you can also try the following combination: Combine
one cup of tart cherry juice with one cup of ACV. Mix them together thoroughly, then add two tablespoons of it to eight ounces of water, refrigerating
the rest of the mixture for later use. Drink two to three glasses per day.

What Else to Consider

To treat arthritis effectively, you need to work with a trained arthritis specialist, preferably one who does not regard your condition as incurable, as so
many conventional doctors do. Ideally, you will want to work with a physician with a background in dietary intervention, nutritional medicine, and
detoxification.

ASTHMA

Asthma can be either chronic or short-term, and in some cases an acute attack
of asthma may require hospitalization. Asthma is caused when the smooth
muscles that surround air passages into the lungs (the bronchi and bronchi-
oles) begin to spasm. Once spasms occur, the bronchial passages narrow, making it more difficult to breathe. During asthma attacks, excessive mucus
production can also occur, further blocking the bronchial passages.

Symptoms

Individuals suffering from asthma may experience an inflammation of the bronchial tubes which results in shortness of breath, a tightness or pressure in the chest, a buildup of mucus, coughing, and/or wheezing.

Causes

Asthma can be caused by a variety of factors, ranging from food allergies, environmental toxins, dust, pollen, dander, mold, exposure to cigarette smoke, exposure to chemicals, poor diet, and nutritional deficiencies. Stress, cold temperatures, and physical over-exertion can also trigger asthma attacks.

Benefits

Apple cider vinegar can help relieve asthma symptoms because of its natural antihistamine effects, as well as because of its acid-alkaline balancing properties, and its ability to thin mucus. You can use ACV in three ways to help minimize asthma symptoms: As a tonic, as part of a steam treatment, and as a bath soak.

ACV Treatment

To use as a *tonic,* combine one to two tablespoons of ACV with eight ounces of pure, filtered water. Drink one to three glasses per day.

To make a *steam* treatment, add one cup of ACV to a pan, along with four to six cups of water. Bring the water to a boil. Once this happens, turn off the stove and cover your head with a towel, deeply inhaling the steam from the mixture. Don't force your breath and continue to breathe with your head covered until your symptoms lessen.

To prepare an ACV *bath soak,* fill your tub with water as hot as you can tolerate, and add three to four cups of ACV. Soak for 20 to 30 minutes, with your body submerged up to your neck if it is comfortable for you to do so. Inhale deeply as you soak to obtain similar benefits as those of the ACV steam.

What Else to Consider

Because asthma symptoms can be caused by a variety of factors, it is important to work with a respiratory specialist who can help you to best determine the causes affecting you. I also recommend that you avoid mucus-producing foods such as dairy products, sugars, simple carbohydrates, and, of course, all junk foods. Instead, emphasize a diet that includes a plentiful supply of fresh fruits and vegetables (ideally organic if you can afford them), wild caught fish, free-range poultry, and whole grains, while also drinking plenty of pure, filtered water each day.

BACK PAIN

Back pain, a discomfort in the back that may become disabling, is one of the most common health problems in the United States; the second leading cause of doctor visits. In addition, the third most common surgery performed in the U.S. is back surgery.

Symptoms

Even though there are a variety of factors that may cause back pain, most often the symptoms are similar. The pain can stretch in intensity from mild to severe. One may experience:

- Aches, stiffness, or tenderness along the back muscles
- Chronic ache or pain in middle or lower back
- Inability to stand straight
- Localized, sharp pain in the neck, upper back, or lower back
- Muscle spasms in lower back
- Pain radiating from lower back to buttock
- Pain shooting down leg (numbness)

Causes

There are various causes of back pain, many of which are physical and structural in nature. These range from injuries and tears of muscles, tendons, ligaments and joints, fractures, herniated and degenerative discs, spinal misalignments (subluxations), and, muscle spasms and strains, scoliosis, and imbalances in the pelvis, knees, or feet. Inflammation can also cause back pain, as can arthritis, chronic stress, and a sedentary lifestyle.

Nutritional deficiencies, including potassium, which is found in ACV, can also cause or contribute to back pain because of how these deficiencies can trigger muscle tightness and lactic acid buildup, along with impair circulation within muscle tissues.

Benefits

While apple cider vinegar is most definitely not a cure for back pain, it can help to reduce the severity of back pain symptoms.

ACV Treatment

Taken as a *tonic* (one to two tablespoons of ACV added to eight ounces of pure, filtered water), it can help to reduce inflammation. A hot apple cider vinegar *bath soak* (four to six cups of ACV added to hot bath water) can further soothe and relax muscles that are tight or spasming. You can soak in such baths for 30 minutes or more.

What Else to Consider

Since back pain is primarily a physical, structural problem, it is important that you work with a skilled, health professional who knows how to accurately diagnose and treat back pain's underlying causes. Such professionals include chiropractors, bodyworkers, physical and occupational therapists, and osteopathic physicians who do not rely on drugs or surgery as primary forms of back pain treatment.

Acupuncture treatments can also be helpful, as can learning how to effectively exercise, including performing stretching exercises. (If you are unused to regular exercise, start slowly and consider initially working with a professional trainer.)

Persistent back pain located in the mid- to outer areas of the mid- or lower back can sometimes be an indicator of kidney stones. If you suspect you are suffering from kidney stones, consult your physician who will most likely schedule an x-ray or other diagnostic test for you.

See also **KIDNEY PROBLEMS.**

BAD BREATH (HALITOSIS)

Bad breath, or halitosis, affects nearly everyone at some point in their lives. For most people, the most common form of bad breath is "morning breath," which occurs during sleep and is present upon awakening.

Symptoms

The odors associated with halitosis vary depending upon the origin of the underlying cause. Besides a bad smell in your mouth, you may also observe a bad taste in your mouth.

Causes

Bad breath usually results from bacteria in the mouth, which, in turn, can be due to poor dietary habits, failure to adequately take care of one's teeth and gums, or lifestyle habits such as smoking. It can also be a result of other health problems, such as a sinus infection, chronic postnasal drip, diabetes, and acid reflux disease.

Benefits

To help prevent bad breath, it is important that you follow proper dental hygiene, including regular brushing of your teeth and flossing of your gums. Gargling with a mouthwash can also be helpful. Unfortunately, most commercial mouthwashes contain a variety of ingredients that aren't safe if swallowed. Apple cider vinegar in the form of a gargle or mouth rinse offers a safe and effective alternative.

ACV is helpful for preventing bad breath because of its antibacterial and antiseptic properties, making it an ideal natural solution for treating bacteria on your teeth, gums, and tongue.

ACV Treatment

Making an apple cider vinegar *mouthwash or rinse* is very easy. Simply combine on tablespoon of ACV with half a cup of pure, filtered water. Mix thoroughly, then swish or gargle in your mouth for 30 to 60 seconds, then spit the mixture out. Repeat as necessary. For best results, do this after you first brush your teeth, and floss your gums in the morning and before going to bed. (Do not swish or gargle with apple cider vinegar that is not diluted in water. Because of its acidic content undiluted ACV can potentially harm the enamel of your teeth.)

What Else to Consider

If you suffer from chronic bad breath, please consult with your dentist, as this could be a sign of an underlying gum condition, such as gingivitis. Chronic bad breath can sometimes also indicate sinus infection, or infection in the tonsils or lungs. In some cases, bad breath can also be a sign of impaired digestion (especially of proteins) or other gastrointestinal problems.

BLADDER PROBLEMS

Bladder problems can vary widely, ranging from infections (especially E. coli strains) in the urinary tract (UTIs), pain in the bladder or ureter, inflammation of the bladder (bladder cystitis), or uremia (blood in the urine). In men, difficulty urinating or frequent urination can also occur with aging due to the enlargement of the prostate gland.

Symptoms

A bladder problem may be characterized by the following common symptoms:

- Bloody or cloudy urine
- Burning or pain during urination
- Fever and chills, when severe

- Foul-smelling urine
- Pressure or cramping in lower back or abdomen
- Urge to urinate frequently

Causes

Bladder problems may be caused by a variety of factors, including:

- Age, the elderly
- Diabetes
- Difficulty emptying bladder
- Enlarged prostate

- Immobility
- Insufficient fluid intake
- Pregnancy
- Urinary blockage

Benefits

For bladder problems caused by bacterial infections apple cider vinegar can often provide some degree of relief. Once again, this is primarily due to ACV's antiseptic and antibacterial properties. According to noted health expert Earl Mindell, Ph.D, ACV can also help to prevent and possibly even reverse bladder infections because of its ability to increase the acidity within the environment of the bladder and urinary tract, along with the acidity of the urine. This, in turn, helps to prevent and reverse bacterial overgrowth.

ACV Treatment

If you suffer from infection-related bladder problems, try drinking glasses of apple cider vinegar *tonic* throughout the day. Simply mix one or two tablespoons of ACV with eight ounces of pure, filtered water and drink this mixture four or more times each day.

Soaking in a *hot bath* can also help soothe bladder problems by helping to relax the bladder and ureter muscles. For added benefit, you can add four cups of ACV to your bath and soak for 20 to 30 minutes.

What Else to Consider

Persistent bladder problems lasting more than a few days can lead to more serious health problems. Therefore, if your problem persists, seek immediate medical attention. To help prevent bladder problems, be sure to eat a healthy diet and drink plenty of pure, filtered water throughout each day. For more information on why diet and adequate water intake are so important *see* Chapter 5.

See also **URINARY TRACT INFECTIONS.**

BLOOD PRESSURE ISSUES

There are two types of blood pressure conditions: high blood pressure (hypertension) and low blood pressure (hypotension). Both conditions can be serious and, if persistent, require immediate medical attention. Of the two, high blood pressure is more prevalent and more serious, as persistent high blood pressure can lead to heart attack and stroke.

Symptoms

A normal, healthy blood pressure reading is typically lower than 120/80 mm Hg. High blood pressure occurs when a reading is above this level, while low pressure is evident if a reading is significantly below this level. However, your blood pressure isn't always the same, and can vary considerably even within a short amount of time due to a variety of factors, such as your stress levels, your body position, and your breath rate and the fullness of your breath. Other health conditions can also affect blood pressure levels, as can what you eat and drink, various medications you may be on, and whether you have been physically active or sedentary before a blood pressure reading is taken. Overall, blood pressure is usually lowest at night and then noticeably increases in the morning when you wake.

Causes

Many factors can contribute to both high and low blood pressure levels. They range from poor diet, nutritional imbalances and deficiencies, chronic low level dehydration, lack of exercise, other poor lifestyle choices, such as smoking and excessive alcohol consumption, and exposure to environmental toxins. Hardening of the arteries (atherosclerosis) is another common cause of high blood pressure.

Benefits

While apple cider vinegar is certainly not a cure for either high or low blood pressure, it can be helpful as an aid in regulating blood pressure levels. One reason for why ACV can help stabilize blood pressure levels has to do with its pectin content. As you learned in Chapter 2, pectin is a type of soluble fiber that has been shown to help protect against high cholesterol by lowering LDL (so-called "bad") cholesterol and to help reduce high blood pressure levels. As you also learned in Chapter 2, apple cider vinegar also contains potassium, an essential mineral nutrient for regulating blood pressure levels.

Yet it is likely that it is ACV's acetic acid content that is most responsible for ACV's ability to help manage blood pressure levels. This conclusion can be drawn from a number of animal studies that have demonstrated acetic acid's ability in this regard. In the studies, all of which involved hypertensive rats, various vinegars, all of which contain acetic acid, were administered to the rats. The studies found that the acetic acid in the vinegars reduced both plasma renin activity and plasma aldosterone levels in the rats by as much as 40 and 25 percent, respectively. Both plasma renin activity and plasma aldosterone levels are factors that can cause blood vessels to constrict, thus elevating blood pressure levels. The studies also found that the use of vinegar helped prevent the activity of a substance known as angiotension-converting enzyme (ACE) in the rats. ACE can cause high blood pressure by causing blood vessels to become constricted. One of the common medications used in the treatment of high blood pressure are known as ACE-inhibitors. These drugs are not without the risk of serious side effects. ACV, on the other, is perfectly safe and provides some degree of the same benefits as the drugs do.

ACV Treatment

Although no studies have yet been conducted to see if acetic acid and vinegar can produce the same benefits in humans suffering from high blood pressure, Patricia Bragg reports that many of her clients have improved their blood pressure levels and overall health by drinking one or more apple cider vinegar drinks, along with other lifestyle changes similar to what I shared in with you in Chapter 5. Given ACV's safety it makes sense to try and see if drinking an apple cider vinegar *tonic* can improve your blood pressure levels as well. To do so, simply drink one or two glasses of ACV *tonic* each day (one to two tablespoons of ACV added to eight ounces of pure, filtered water).

What Else to Consider

If you suffer from persistent blood pressure problems you need to consult with your doctor. He or she can help determine the underlying causes that are contributing to your problem, and prescribe a proper treatment program for you. Ideally, you should work with a physician trained in integrative or functional medicine, so that he or she can properly evaluate your diet, nutritional status, lifestyle, and other factors that may be associated with your problem.

BLOOD SUGAR ISSUES

Like blood pressure, there are two main types of blood sugar conditions, high blood sugar (hyperglycemia) and low blood sugar (hypoglycemia). Both conditions, if left untreated, can lead to more serious health issues. While both conditions are also associated with diabetes, low blood sugar can also be an indication of adrenal stress and problems in the pancreas, among other conditions. Of the two conditions, most people who suffer from blood sugar problems have high blood sugar, also known as glucose. Persistent blood sugar issues require immediate medical attention.

Symptoms

Hyperglycemia or high blood sugar is a condition where one experiences an increased thirst and a frequent need to urinate. Hypoglycemia or low blood sugar may display early signs such as:

- Confusion
- Dizziness
- Feeling shaky
- Headaches
- Pounding heart, racing pulse
- Sweating

Causes

Blood sugar levels often fluctuate depending on the foods and beverages a person consumes. In order to regulate blood sugar levels after meals, your body requires insulin, a hormone that is critical for the overall regulation of blood glucose levels. Each time that you eat, the foods you consume are broken down into glucose, your body's primary fuel source. Glucose then enters your bloodstream. As it does so, your pancreas, the organ responsible for insulin production, produces insulin to ensure that proper blood glucose levels are maintained. Insulin does this by clearing away excess glucose from the bloodstream, sending it into the liver, where it is converted into glycogen to be used as fuel for your muscles. Any leftover glucose is converted into fatty acids by insulin and stored in fat cells.

Due to the standard American diet, as well as the overconsumption of both simple and complex carbohydrates, many people today are developing what is known as insulin resistance, a condition in which the body can't respond properly to the insulin it produces. As a result, over time, blood sugar levels begin to rise beyond levels that are healthy, potentially leading to diabetes and other metabolic disorders.

Benefits

Numerous studies dating back to 1988 have demonstrated that apple cider vinegar, as well as other vinegars, have a positive effect on the human body's insulin response and help to lower blood glucose levels after meals, primarily due to its acetic acid content. In one of these studies, 29 human test subjects, some of whom were pre-diabetic, were given two tablespoons of apple cider vinegar prior to consuming a high starch meal consisting of a bagel and orange juice. A control group was also fed the same meal, without first consuming ACV. The blood sugar levels of both groups were tested one hour after the meal. Compared to the control group, all of the 29 people showed significantly reduced blood sugar levels, with the pre-diabetic subjects having their blood sugar levels reduced to less than half of the pre-diabetics in the control group. Other studies have further confirmed the ability of ACV and other vinegars to reduce blood glucose levels after meals while also improving the body's insulin response.

Additional research has shown that the acetic acid in ACV and other vinegars can actually reduce the glycemic index (GI) of foods. The glycemic index indicates the effects of a particular food on blood sugar levels. The higher the glycemic index of a food is, the more that food will cause a spike in blood sugar levels after it is consumed. Researchers in Japan, for example, found that taking vinegar with white rice, which has a high glycemic index, can reduce the rice's GI by as much as 35 percent. Subsequent research has shown that vinegar taken before or with meals can reduce the glycemic index of breads and other starches by an average of 30 percent. Research has also shown that consuming vinegar before bedtime can also reduce blood glucose levels during the night.

One of the leading researchers into the health properties of apple cider vinegar is Carol S. Johnston, Ph.D, R.D., Professor and Associate Director of the Nutrition Program in the School of Nutrition and Health Promotion at Arizona State University. Dr. Johnston reports that the acetic acid in ACV and other vinegars prevents a percentage of starchy, high GI foods from being digested and raising blood sugar levels, adding that its effects are similar in nature to blood sugar medications.

ACV Treatment

There are a number of ways that you can use ACV to improve blood sugar levels. The first is to consume a glass of ACV and pure, filtered water before meals, especially meals that contain starchy foods. You can also marinate both raw and steamed vegetable with ACV, and use it as a dressing on salads.

What Else to Consider

ACV alone is unlikely to address persistent blood sugar problems. If you suffer from such problems, please see your doctor. In addition, pay attention to your diet, avoiding sugar and sugary food and beverages, and limit your intake of carbohydrate and other high glycemic foods. (To quickly and easily determine the glycemic index of foods and beverages, visit the website www.glycemicindex.com, a free online resource provided by the University of Sidney, Australia.)

BODY ODOR

Body odor affects all of us from time to time, and some people sweat more or less than others. Sweating, which may result in body odor, can occur when you exercise, when you're too warm, when you're nervous, anxious, or under stress.

Causes

Body odor is most commonly caused by dried sweat on the skin for a few hours, especially sweat located under and around the armpits. During this time, skin bacteria decompose the sweat, in some cases causing an unpleasant body odor. Unpleasant body odor can be prevented or at least significantly minimized by healthy hygiene practices, including showering or bathing on a daily basis.

Benefits

Most people in America today also use some type of deodorant or antiperspirant to prevent body odor. While such products can be effective, commercial deodorants and antiperspirants are not without health risks. Both can contain a variety of potentially unsafe chemicals, including artificial fragrances, aluminum, parabens, and various petrochemicals, all of which can be toxic when absorbed into the skin. (Aluminum, for instance, has been linked to both dementia and Alzheimer's disease, while parabens, petrochemicals, and certain ingredients that make up artificial fragrances have all been linked to cancer.) Moreover, antiperspirants work by literally clogging up armpit pores, preventing them from allowing sweat to pass through the skin from inside the body, as nature intended. Fortunately, apple cider vinegar offers a safe, effective, and very inexpensive alternative to store-bought deodorants and antiperspirants.

ACV Treatment

Simply add equal parts of ACV and water together and mix thoroughly. Then, after showering or bathing, use a cotton ball or a cotton cloth soaked with the mixture and apply it under your armpits and then allow the mixture to dry.

What Else to Consider

Certain foods, such as garlic and onions, can contribute to unpleasant body odor. Body odor that persists can also be due to nutritional deficiencies (especially zinc), as well as liver dysfunction and toxicity, and/or gastrointestinal problems, such as constipation. If body odor persists, consult your doctor to screen for such underlying conditions. Also be sure to keep your body clean via a daily shower or bath.

BONE LOSS (OSTEOPOROSIS)

Bone loss, also known as osteoporosis, is an increasingly common occurrence among people in the U.S. and other Western industrialized countries as they age, especially among women as they enter or pass through menopause. Some people, with a family history of the disorder, are genetically prone to it. A medical condition or treatment may trigger the condition as well.

Symptoms

Early symptoms of bone loss or weakened bones are:

- Back pain
- Bone fracture

- Shrinking, loss of height over a period of time
- Stooped posture

Causes

Bone loss is primarily due to the acidifying effects of the diets most people in these countries follow. (By comparison, cultures around the world that follow a diet consisting of primarily alkalizing foods have virtually no incidence of osteoporosis in their populations, nor of most other chronic, degenerative diseases that are so common in the U.S., Canada, and Europe, including heart disease and cancer.) Bone loss can also be caused by other factors, as well, including lack of exercise (particularly strength training exercises), hormonal imbalances, smoking, and the use of pharmaceutical drugs.

As bone loss occurs, calcium, magnesium, potassium, and other minerals are displaced from the bones into other parts of the body. Not only does this weaken bones and cause them to become more porous, and thus more prone to fracture and breaking, in the case of calcium it can also lead to calcium deposits in the arteries and kidneys. A diet that is high in acidifying, rather than alkalizing, food and beverages hasten this process. In order to neutralize acid buildup in its tissues and organs, the body pulls the above mentioned mineral, all of which are acid-neutralizers, out of the bones to quench the "acid fires" caused by such foods.

Benefits

While apple cider vinegar, by itself, cannot entirely prevent bone loss, and certainly not reverse it, ACV can help to reduce the risk of bone loss in two ways. First, as you've already learned, when ACV is consumed it has an overall alkalizing effect in the body. Second, as I mentioned in Chapter 2, the acetic and other acids ACV contains can help to improve your body's ability to more fully absorb and make use of the wide array of nutrients that you consume each day in your food, acting in much the same way that enzymes do. With regard to bone loss, this is important because calcium, magnesium, and potassium are often poorly absorbed, both when obtained from foods, and in the form of nutritional supplements.

ACV Treatment

By including ACV as part of your daily diet, as well as eating a diet that contains a plentiful supply of mineral-rich foods, you will help your body better absorb and make use of the nutrients it needs, both for maintaining the health of your bones, and for the literally hundreds of other uses.

Introduce ACV into your diet as a *tonic* in water (one tablespoon of ACV added to eight ounces of pure, filtered water) once or twice a day and as a *dressing* on salads and on raw and steamed vegetables.

What Else to Consider

If you suspect you suffer from bone loss, consult with your doctor. He or she can confirm whether or not you are experiencing bone loss by measuring your bone density. One of the most effective and accurate means of doing so is through the use of a DXA (dual X-ray absorptiometry) test, which has a 99 percent accuracy rate. This is the test I recommend you ask for, instead of a simple X-ray or CT scan. You should also work with your doctor or a certified clinical nutritionist to assess health of your diet and to determine what nutritional deficiencies you may have.

BRUISING

Bruising is typically caused by injury. A bruise or contusion may result after a cut or blow to the skin, when you bump into something, or when you exercise strenuously.

Symptoms

Usually bruises initially appear as black or blue, then, as the healing process progresses, bruises begin to lighten, turning yellowish before fading away altogether.

Causes

When an injury occurs, blood below the surface of the injury site leaks out of capillaries to collect beneath the injury site causing temporary discoloration on the skin.

Benefits

Although most bruises will heal on their own, you can use an apple cider vinegar compress to help speed up the healing process. ACV helps to heal bruising because, when applied to the bruise area, the acids, enzymes, and nutrients it contains help to cleanse and nourish the skin.

ACV Treatment

Making an apple cider vinegar *compress* is easy. Simply soak a clean washcloth with ACV and hold it over the bruised area for a few minutes, allowing the ACV to penetrate into the skin. You can repeat this process a few times each day until your bruise disappears.

What Else to Consider

Bruising that persists or recurs can be a sign of an underlying health problem. A lack of vitamin C and other nutritional deficiencies can result in slower than normal healing of bruises. Persistent bruising can also be an indication of bleeding disorders. If you experience persistent or recurring bruising, seek immediate medical attention.

BURNS

While serious burns require immediate medical attention, minor first degree burns in which only the outer surface area of the skin is affected will typically heal on their own within a few days or more.

Symptoms

First degree burns generate pain and reddening of the skin (the outer layer). Second degree burns cause swelling, pain, blistering, and redness and affects the outer and lower layer of the skin. Third degree burns result in charred skin that may feel numb and affects deeper tissues.

Causes

A burn is damage to your body's skin that may be brought about by extreme heat or cold, chemicals, electricity, sunlight, or radiation. In a first degree burn, the skin will redden and may peel away as part of the healing process. Should you suffer such a burn, immediately run cold water over the site of your injury and keep doing so for up to 30 minutes or more. This will help ease the pain and can also help to prevent blistering. Once you finish running cold water, gently dry the area.

Benefits

There are a number of reasons why apple cider vinegar can aid in the healing of minor burns. First, as Hippocrates taught many centuries ago, ACV is very effective for protecting against infections, and thus able to prevent harmful bacteria and other microbes from attacking the burn area. Second, the acids and nutrients ACV contains can assist your skins ability to repair itself. Finally, the compounds in ACV can help to reduce inflammation and minimize swelling around the burn area.

ACV Treatment

You can make an apple cider vinegar *bandage* to apply over the burn area. To do so, combine a quarter cup of ACV with one cup of cool water. Mix thoroughly, then soak gauze in the mixture. Remove the gauze and squeeze out the excess moisture, then apply it over the burn site, holding it in place with bandaging. Reapply a new ACV-soaked gauze *bandage* once a day until the burn site is fully healed.

What Else to Consider

If you are uncertain as to the degree of your burn, seek prompt medical attention. You should also seek medical attention if your burn shows little to no sign of healing within a few days.

CALLUSES

Calluses are thick, hardened areas of skin that form as a result of repeated pressure, friction, some other type of irritation to the affected area. Writers, for example, can sometimes develop calluses on their fingers if they regularly write with a pen or pencil, and calluses are also common among musicians who play string instruments, especially guitar, bass, and violin.

Symptoms

The appearance of calluses include:

- Dry flaky skin
- Raised hardened patch of skin
- Tenderness or pain in the area
- Thick or hard or rough area of skin

Causes

The repeated pressure, friction, or irritation to the skin causes the skin to die and create a hard, protective surface. The most common areas of the body in which calluses form are the feet and toes, although they can also form on fingers. Overall, while they can be unsightly, calluses are not harmful and require no medical attention.

Benefits

Regularly using ACV soaks to treat calluses will help to further soften them, while simultaneously improving circulation and relieving inflammation.

ACV Treatment

A common self-care treatment for calluses is to rub them with pumice stones. Doing so over time helps to break down hardened skin. To improve this method, you can also use an apple cider vinegar *soak*. To make an ACV *soak*, add one to two cups of ACV to enough bath water to cover your feet. The water should be hot but tolerable. Then sit on the edge of your bath or in a chair, and soak your feet in this solution for 20 to 30 minutes a day. If sitting over a bath is not feasible for you, you can add the ACV and hot water to a pan large enough to soak both of your feet in at once. A smaller pan can also be used for soaking calluses on your fingers.

Prior to the *soak*, treating your calluses with a pumice stone to soften them will help the ACV solution to better penetrate into the calluses. Once you complete your *soak*, you can, if you wish, apply another pumice stone treatment after you dry your feet or hands. Doing so will further eliminate dead skin from calluses.

What Else to Consider

Although the vast majority of cases of calluses are harmless, in some instances they can become infected or lead to skin ulcerations. If this happens, seek prompt medical attention. Since calluses that form on the feet and toes are often caused by the shoes people wear, if you suffer from persistent calluses on your feet or toes you may wish to consult with a podiatrist who can prescribe more appropriate and comfortable footwear. I also recommend going barefoot as much as possible when you can, as doing so will help your feet and toes to release constriction.

See also CORNS.

CANDIDIASIS (CANDIDA)

Candidiasis, also known simply as candida, is systemic disease caused by the overgrowth of yeast, specifically the yeast called *Candida albicans* (hence its name). Candida albicans exists in all of us and is part of the various intestinal flora that harmlessly reside in the lower intestinal tract, on our skin, and, in women, within the vagina. In healthy individuals, Candida and other potentially harmful flora are kept in check by a variety of healthy bacteria that also inhabit the human body. But when the balance between healthy bacteria and other flora becomes disrupted, Candida growth increases. As it does so, Candida can transform from a harmless, simple form of yeast into a more aggressive yeast fungus capable of spreading beyond where it normally occurs in and on the body, entering the blood stream to create a systemic infection. This is candidiasis.

Symptoms

Candidiasis is sometimes referred to as a "stealth disease" because of how varied its symptoms can be, leading many sufferers and their physicians to mistake it for other health conditions. The most common symptoms of candidiasis are:

- Allergies
- Anxiety and irritability
- "Brain fog" and memory loss
- Chronic, unexplained fatigue
- Depression
- Headache and migraine
- Heart palpitations
- Mood swings
- Rashes and hives
- Recurring and persistent fungal infections, including athletes' foot and "jock itch"
- Respiratory problems
- Sinus problems
- Sleep problems
- Stomach bloating and other gastrointestinal disturbances, such as diarrhea, constipation, and intestinal cramps
- Unexplained weight gain

Because of the wide range of symptoms candidiasis can cause, it can often go un- or misdiagnosed for years. Fortunately, various blood tests as well as a stool analysis can detect candidiasis, so if you suspect you have it, ask your doctor to provide you with such tests.

Causes

Systemic candida infections most commonly strike people who eat a diet high in sugars, simple carbohydrates, and processed foods, people who suffer from nutritional deficiencies, people with a weakened immune system, people who regularly use broad spectrum antibiotic drugs (these kill off healthy flora in the GI tract), people who excessively consume alcohol (especially beer, which contains yeast), people with hormonal imbalances, and women who use birth control pills or who have undergone synthetic estrogen replacement therapy.

Benefits

Because candidiasis *is* a systemic health condition, a comprehensive treatment plan is usually necessary in order to fully resolve it. This can include prescription drugs such as Nystatin, if necessary, along with an anti-candida diet, proper nutritional supplementation, and, if appropriate, herbal medicine.

Apple cider vinegar can often enhance the effectiveness of such treatments when consumed as an ACV tonic or applied topically to fungal overgrowth caused by Candida yeast. ACV's benefits for treating candidiasis derive from the acetic acid and natural enzymes it contains, all of which can help regulate the growth of Candida yeast in the body. Additionally, apple cider vinegar also helps check Candida overgrowth because of its overall alkalizing effects when it is consumed. Like all other types of harmful microbes, the Candida yeast thrives in an overly acidic environment. Regular consumption of ACV in water helps to raise the pH level of such environments. Additionally, once consumed, apple cider vinegar acts as a healthy prebiotic, stimulating the growth of healthy bacteria in your gut that can further bring unhealthy flora back in check.

ACV Treatment

To augment an overall candidiasis treatment plan, I recommend drinking three glasses of apple cider vinegar *tonic* each day, ideally 20 minutes or more before breakfast, lunch, and dinner. For each glass, add one tablespoon of ACV to eight ounces of pure, filtered water, or you can try filling a water bottle with ACV and water and sip it throughout the day.

If you suffer from external signs of candidiasis, such as fungal infections, you can apply apple cider vinegar *topically* over the affected areas. Unless you have sensitive skin, there is no need to dilute the ACV. You can also *soak* in an ACV bath. Simply add three to four cups of ACV to a comfortable, hot bath and soak for 20 to 30 minutes once a day.

What Else to Consider

To properly treat candidiasis, you need to work with a health professional who knows how to most effectively deal with it. You also need to strictly adhere to an anti-Candida diet. This means eliminating all sugars, simple carbohydrates, starchy foods, processed foods, alcohol, and even fruits with a high glycemic index, high sugar content (visit the website www.glycemicindex.com, a free online resource provided by the University of Sidney, Australia, to quickly and easily determine the glycemic index of the foods and beverages you consume.) Emphasize a diet of fresh, low, starchy vegetables, fresh, low sugar fruits, free range poultry and meats and wild caught fish, along with raw nuts and seeds. Fermented foods, such as sauerkraut, miso, and kimchi are also recommended since they also act as natural prebiotics.

Also note that, once you begin your treatment for candidiasis, you may initially begin to feel worse than before you did so. This is a natural reaction known as the Herxheimer reaction, and is caused by the Candida yeast dying off. As the yeast die, they release toxic byproducts and waste matter that cause nausea, fatigue, headache, and various other symptoms. In most cases, these symptoms will subside within a few days to a few weeks, depending on the severity of your condition. After that, you should experience steady, noticeable improvement.

See also **YEAST INFECTIONS.**

CHOLESTEROL

Cholesterol is a naturally occurring and most common type of steroid in the body steroid. Although most people think of cholesterol as a risk factor for heart disease, in actuality it is vitally important to our health. Not only is it essential for the production of numerous hormones, including estrogens, testosterone, progesterone, and cortisol, among others, without cholesterol our bodies could not produce vitamin D and the various bile acids that are necessary for the proper digestion of dietary fats. Just as important, cholesterol protects all of the body's nerves, and is essential for maintaining proper functioning of the membranes that surround and protect our bodies' cells, as well as for maintaining cellular membrane permeability. While a certain amount of cholesterol enters the body through the foods we eat, especially foods high in saturated fats, the most cholesterol in the body is produced by the liver.

Symptoms

An elevated cholesterol level generally does not display any symptoms. Usually, it can lead to life threatening emergencies, such as a stroke or heart attack.

Causes (High Cholesterol)

While for decades, starting in the 1950s, elevated cholesterol levels were demonized as a primary cause of heart disease, in recent years researchers have discovered that it is not cholesterol by itself that is to blame, but whether or not the cholesterol becomes oxidized due to inflammation, bacterial overload, and an overly acidic diet. Lifestyle factors such as smoking and being overweight can also cause cholesterol to become oxidized because of the inflammation they both cause. When cholesterol becomes oxidized, it can cause atherosclerosis (hardening of the arteries), a significant precursor condition for both heart disease and stroke.

For improved health, it is wise to maintain healthy HDL (high-density), LDL (low-density, also known as bad cholesterol), and total levels. According to the National Institutes of Health (NIH), optimal cholesterol levels are:

- LDL—less than 100 mg/dl
- HDL—60 mg/dl and above
- Total cholesterol—less than 200 mg/dl.

Your doctor can quickly and easily determine your cholesterol levels with a simple blood test, and it is a good idea to monitor your cholesterol on a regular basis, such as an annual health checkup. When doing so, also ask that your levels of C-reactive protein (CRP) and homocysteine levels be checked, as both of these are markers for inflammation.

Benefits

There is much that you can do on your own to maintain and, if necessary, lower your cholesterol levels, including eating a healthy diet and engaging in regular exercise (*see* Chapter 5), as well as losing weight if you need to do so, and not smoking. In addition, you can also use apple cider vinegar.

The cholesterol-lowering effects of apple cider vinegar, acetic acid, its main component, and polyphenols, which ACV also contains, have been proven by scientific research. Numerous human epidemiological studies (studies that analyze patterns, causative factors, and their effects on the health of and incidence of disease within defined populations), have clearly established that populations that follow diets that contain a plentiful supply of polyphenol-rich foods have a significantly lower risk of heart disease and other conditions, and also tend to live longer. A good example of this can be found in cultures that follow the Mediterranean diet. Similar studies have also shown that polyphenols, such as those found in apple cider vinegar, can help decrease the formation of oxidized LDL cholesterol in the bloodstream and thus reduce the risk of heart disease.

A number of animal studies have also demonstrated the ability of acetic acid to reduce both levels of total and LDL cholesterol and triglycerides (another risk factor for heart disease), including in rats fed a high cholesterol diet while also receiving apple cider vinegar, while also increasing good HDL cholesterol levels. More significantly, a human study of 19 men and women, all of whom presented with hyperlipidemia (a condition of elevated, unhealthy fats and cholesterol in the bloodstream), clearly found apple cider vinegar has benefit as a cholesterol-lowering agent. All of the patients had total cholesterol levels greater than 200 mg/dL and/or triglyceride levels greater than 150 mg/dL, both of which are indications of heart disease risk.

According to the researchers who conducted the study, "At the beginning of the study, blood lipids of eligible individuals were tested. All participants were asked not to modify their diet or physical activity pattern. However, they had to consume 30 ml of apple cider vinegar, 4 percent, twice a day (morning and afternoon) for eight weeks. At the end of the second, fourth, and eighth weeks, 5 ml blood samples were obtained after 14 hours of fasting. Cholesterol, triglyceride, HDL, and LDL levels were then determined using enzymatic methods in the laboratory."

At the end of the study, it was found that the patients' total cholesterol, LDL, and triglycerides levels all had significantly been reduced, with total cholesterol reduction being at similar levels for all of the study participants. (The reduction in LDL levels was most noticeable in men, while in women the reduction of triglycerides was most pronounced.) Based on the results of this study, the researchers wrote," In general, the present study indicated that consumption of apple cider vinegar can reduce the LDL, triglyceride, and cholesterol levels in patients with hyperlipidemia. Besides, given that hyper-lipidemia is a known risk factor for atherosclerosis, apple cider vinegar can be used to prevent and even treat this complication and probably other heart problems."

ACV Treatment

To obtain similar benefits as the study participants in the study received from apple cider vinegar, consider drinking one or two glasses of ACV *tonic* each day, combining one tablespoon of ACV to eight ounces of pure, filtered water.

What Else to Consider

If you suffer from high cholesterol you would be foolish to rely on ACV alone to resolve your problem. You also need to follow a healthy diet, engage in regular exercise, avoid unhealthy lifestyle habits, such as smoking and excessive alcohol consumption, and, if necessary, lose weight. Also work with your doctor and be sure to be screened regularly (at least once a year) using blood tests to monitor your cholesterol levels and levels of inflammation.

See also **WEIGHT LOSS.**

COMMON COLDS

At least half the population of the United States experiences a common cold one or more times each year. Unlike the flu, which is much more serious and can even be life-threatening, the common cold is usually not severe and usually lasts for no more than a few days to a few weeks. While the flu tends to occur seasonally, hence the medical communities focus on the "flu season," colds can occur any time of year.

Symptoms

Colds are not something to look forward to, presenting as they do with:

- Congestion
- Coughs
- Fatigue
- Headache
- Sore throat

Causes

Like flu, colds are caused by respiratory viruses. However, it is not the viruses themselves that determine whether or not you will "catch" a cold. Rather, it depends on the health of your immune system and whether or not your body is in a state of chronic, low-grade acidity due to your diet. Like all other types of viruses, as well as bacteria and fungi, cold viruses thrive in an overly acidic environment within the body.

Benefits

It is because of these two factors that apple cider vinegar can prove very effective for preventing and speeding recovery from the common cold. First, the acids and nutrients contained in ACV all have immune-enhancing, antiviral properties. Second, when taken orally, apple cider vinegar has an alkalizing effect within the body, meaning it helps neutralize acid buildup.

ACV Treatment

To improve your resistance to the common cold, I recommend that you drink at least one glass of apple cider vinegar *tonic* (one to two tablespoons of ACV added to eight ounces of pure, filtered water) per day. Should you develop a cold, drinking three or four glasses of ACV *tonic* per day will help even more. Doing so will help boost your body's immune function and improve its acid-alkaline balance. In addition, the tonic drink will help ease any congestion associated with your cold due to ACV's ability to thin mucus.

To ease congestion associated with colds, you can also use ACV as a *steam treatment* and in your bath. To make a *steam treatment,* add one cup of ACV to a pan, along with four to six cups of water. Bring the water to a boil. Once this happens, turn off the stove and cover your head with a towel, deeply inhaling the steam from the mixture. Don't force your breath and continue to breathe with your head covered until your symptoms lessen.

To prepare an ACV *bath soak,* fill your tub with water as hot as you can tolerate, and add three to four cups of ACV. Soak for 20 to 30 minutes, with your body submerged up to your neck if it is comfortable for you to do so. Inhale deeply as you soak to obtain similar benefits as those of the ACV steam.

What Else to Consider

To prevent and speed up recovery from a cold avoid mucus-producing foods, such as dairy products, sugars, simple carbohydrates, and, of course, all junk foods. Instead, emphasize a diet that includes a plentiful supply of fresh fruits and vegetables (ideally organic if you can afford them), wild caught fish, free-range poultry, and whole grains, while also drinking plenty of pure, filtered water each day. If your cold symptoms do not improve within a few days or more, it could be a sign of a more serious condition. For persistent colds and colds that recur often, seek prompt medical attention.

CONGESTION

Congestion is a condition caused by an abnormal accumulation of fluid in any organ in the body. The fluid is most often mucus, but it can be bile or blood. Congestion conditions of bile and blood require immediate medical attention and are beyond the scope of this book. Mucus congestion most commonly occurs either within the chest or sinuses.

Symptoms

As the congestion in the sinuses or chest develops, it can make breathing more difficult and also trigger coughs, fatigue, sneezing, and headache.

Causes

Sinus and chest congestion are usually brought on by seasonal allergies or bacterial or viral infections.

Benefits

Apple cider vinegar can help relieve symptoms of chest and sinus congestion for the same reasons that ACV can help prevent and relieve colds. The acids and nutrients contained in ACV all have immune-enhancing, antibacterial and antiviral properties. Just as importantly, ACV's ingredients work together to help thin mucus so that the body can rid itself of excess mucus more easily. ACV also acts as a natural anti-inflammatory agent, which can help alleviate inflammation associated with chest and sinus congestion. Finally, apple cider

Nasal Wash

Your nose is an important, yet often overlooked, organ for keeping you healthy. Not only does your nose take in the oxygen you need to stay alive, processing up to 20, 000 liters of air each and every day, it also acts as a first line of defense to filter out airborne contaminants and other particles, protecting your lungs from damage and infection. Your nose is also responsible for helping to keep your lungs and bronchial tubes from becoming too dry. It does this by moisturizing the air you breathe, and warming cold air.

Keeping your nose clean and free of congestion should therefore be an important part of your daily health routine, especially during cold and flu season. Many people use decongestant nasal sprays for this purpose. While they can be helpful, prolonged use of such sprays can be harmful, as they can damage the cilia in the nose that work to keep nasal passages clear. A healthier alternative is to use apple cider vinegar to make your own nasal wash.

Ideally, you want to use a neti pot for this purpose. Neti pots are commonly available at health food stores and drugstores. If you don't have one available, you can also use an eyedropper or a small cup.

To make an ACV nasal wash solution, combine half a teaspoon of ACV (you don't want to use more than this because of ACV's acidic properties) to a cup of warm, pure, filtered water. Then, tilting your head to one side, gently pour a bit of the solution into one nostril, and sniff it up. Doing so will dislodge mucus and nasal debris, which you can then clear by blowing your nose. Repeat this process with your other nostril. Not only will this wash help clear your nostrils, ACV's antibacterial and antiviral properties will also help protect against airborne infections.

If you suffer from chronic or recurring nasal congestion, see your doctor. During times of nasal congestion, avoid mucus-producing foods, such as dairy products, sugars, simple carbohydrates, and, of course, all junk foods. Instead, emphasize a diet that includes a plentiful supply of fresh fruits and vegetables (ideally organic if you can afford them), wild caught fish, free-range poultry, and whole grains, while also drinking plenty of pure, filtered water each day.

vinegar has an alkalizing effect within the body, meaning it helps neutralize the acids that harmful microorganisms thrive within.

ACV Treatment

To help congestion symptoms, drink at least one glass of apple cider vinegar *tonic* (one to two tablespoons of ACV added to eight ounces of pure, filtered water) per day. Drinking three or four glasses of ACV *tonic* per day will help even more.

To further ease congestion symptoms, you can also use ACV as a *steam* treatment and in your bath. To make a *steam* treatment, add one cup of ACV to a pan, along with four to six cups of water. Bring the water to a boil. Once this happens, turn off the stove and cover your head with a towel, deeply inhaling the steam from the mixture. Don't force your breath and continue to breathe with your head covered until your symptoms lessen.

To prepare an ACV *bath soak,* fill your tub with water as hot as you can tolerate, and add three to four cups of ACV. Soak for 20 to 30 minutes, with your body submerged up to your neck if it is comfortable for you to do so. Inhale deeply as you soak to obtain similar benefits as those of the ACV *steam.*

What Else to Consider

To improve your recovery from congestion, avoid mucus-producing foods, such as dairy products, sugars, simple carbohydrates, and, of course, all junk foods. Instead, emphasize a diet that includes a plentiful supply of fresh fruits and vegetables (ideally organic if you can afford them), wild caught fish, free-range poultry, and whole grains, while also drinking plenty of pure, filtered water each day. If your symptoms do not improve within a few days or more, if could be a sign of a more serious condition. For persistent or recurring congestion, seek prompt medical attention.

See also **SINUSITIS and COMMON COLDS.**

CONSTIPATION

Constipation is one of the most common health problems in the United States. While an occasional bout of constipation is usually not something to be alarmed about, chronic constipation can lead to other health issues, ranging from digestive and other gastrointestinal problems, to the buildup of toxins in the body, and impaired absorption of vital nutrients. Left untreated, chronic constipation can also result in chronic inflammatory and autoimmune diseases, ranging from chronic fatigue to rheumatoid arthritis to colitis, and even lower back pain.

Symptoms

For many, constipation means infrequent bowel movements. For others, you may experience:

- Difficulty passing stools (straining)
- Few bowel movements
- Hard or small stools
- Sense of not being able to completely empty stools
- Swollen stomach or stomach pain
- Throwing up

Causes

Constipation can be caused by a variety of factors. These include:

- Chronic low-grade dehydration
- Chronic stress and other emotional upsets
- Food allergies
- Impaired nutrition
- Lack of exercise
- Low thyroid function (hypothyroidism)
- Pharmaceutical drugs, including laxatives
- Poor diet

All of which over time can impair the body's ability to void the bowels on its own.

To avoid or reverse constipation it is important to follow a diet of healthy, nutritious, fiber-rich foods, keep your body adequately hydrated, engage in regular exercise, and avoid eating meals when you are stressed or emotionally upset. Sugar, simple carbohydrates, fried foods, caffeine, and alcohol can also cause or contribute to constipation, and therefore should also be avoided.

Benefits

Apple cider vinegar can also help prevent and relieve constipation symptoms. ACV is able to do this because of its pectin content (pectin acts as a natural fiber). The acetic acid and other acid compounds ACV contains can also help in two ways. First, they act as natural prebiotics, helping stimulate the growth of healthy bacteria in the GI tract that help to keep us regular. In addition, these compounds also act as natural stool softeners, making it easier for stool to be eliminated from the body.

ACV Treatment

If you suffer from constipation, try drinking one to three glasses of apple cider vinegar *tonic* each day (one tablespoon of ACV combined with eight ounces of pure, filtered water).

What Else to Consider

Chronic constipation can be a symptom of a more serious health condition. If your constipation problems persist, seek the help of your doctor.

CORNS

Corns are hardened growths that occur on toes and toe joints. Corns can be quite painful and, like calluses on the feet, they are most often caused by ongoing friction or pressure on the feet, usually due to footwear problems. They have a hard center and may be surrounded by inflamed skin and are smaller than calluses.

Symptoms

Corns can be quite painful, but the pain can vary, sometimes occurring only in response to pressure, while in other cases corn pain can be constant.

Causes

An abnormal development of the feet, such as a hammertoe, can cause a corn to form, as well as any bony projection on the feet. Shoes that are too tight or too short can lead to the formation of skin thickening that may lead to the development of corns.

Benefit

Apple cider vinegar can help soothe corns in much the same way that it can help relieve calluses, in the form of an apple cider soak. Over time, ACV soaks can help to break down hardened skin.

ACV Treatment

To make an ACV *soak,* add one to two cups of ACV to enough bath water to cover your feet. The water should be hot but tolerable. Then sit on the edge of your bath or in a chair, and soak your feet in this solution for 20 to 30 minutes a day. If sitting over a bath is not feasible for you, you can add the ACV and hot water to a pan or pail large enough to soak both of your feet in at once. Regularly using ACV *soaks* to treat corns will help to further soften them while simultaneously improving circulation and relieving inflammation.

What Else to Consider

Although the vast majority of cases of corns are harmless except for the pain they can cause, in some instances they can become infected or lead to skin ulcerations. If this happens, seek prompt medical attention. If you suffer from persistent corns consult with a podiatrist who can pare corns away and prescribe more appropriate and comfortable footwear. I also recommend going barefoot as much as possible when you can, as doing so will help your feet and toes to release constriction.

See also **CALLUSES.**

COUGHS

All of us cough from time to time simply to clear our throats or because our throats are dry. Coughs can also occur when we are exposed to irritants in the environment, such as dust, smoke, pollen, or chemicals. Under such circumstances, coughing will usually be a fleeting experience that quickly passes once exposure to such irritants ends. But coughs can also linger and be due to congestion or infection as our bodies attempt to move mucus (phlegm) out of the lungs.

Symptoms

A cough may be dry and it may discharge mucus. Symptoms that may be present with a cough include chest pain, fever, sinus congestion, and difficulty breathing.

Causes

A respiratory tract infection, such as a cold or flu, is the most common cause of a cough. These are usually caused by a virus. The following can be responsible for the greater number of chronic coughs:

- Allergies
- Asthma
- Bacterial infection
- Chronic bronchitis
- Gastroesophageal reflux disease (GERD)
- Postnasal drip

Benefit

When coughs caused by congestion or infection occur, apple cider vinegar can often help ease them due to its ability to relieve excess mucus buildup. ACV achieves this effect because of its natural antihistamine effects, as well as because of its acid-alkaline balancing properties, and its ability to thin mucus.

ACV Treatment

The quickest and easiest to relieve coughing using ACV is to have a glass of ACV with water. Simply add one to two tablespoons of ACV to eight ounces of pure, filtered water, and drink it slowly.

You can also use apple cider vinegar to make a natural cough syrup. To do so, combine two tablespoons of ACV with two tablespoons of raw, organic honey and mix them together in eight ounces of water. (You may wish to heat the honey first, so that it mixes more easily.) Honey is well-known for its immune-enhancing properties and also acts as a natural expectorant, helping to move mucus out of the lungs.

What Else to Consider

Persistent coughs are a symptom of a more serious underlying health condition, such as cold, flu, asthma, bronchitis, or pneumonia. If you cough does not resolve within a day or two, seek immediate medical attention.

See also COMMON COLDS.

CUTS

Cuts or lacerations are tears in the skin due to an external injury. These wounds may only affect the surface of the skin or may be more serious where they are deep enough to affect the muscles and tendons. Infection is the most serious risk factor for minor cuts, which otherwise will normally heal on their own without the need for medical attention.

Symptoms

Signs and symptoms that a cut may be infected include:

- Drainage, pus coming from the cut
- Fever
- Pain
- Redness
- Swelling
- Warmth in the affected area

Causes

Cuts may occur as a result of a fall, coming into contact with a hard or sharp object, or being cut by something sharp.

Benefits

As you learned in Chapter 1, Hippocrates, the father of Western medicine, used and wrote of apple cider vinegar's proven benefits to improve wound healing by preventing infection, and right up through World War One, armies went to battle carrying supplies of ACV for this very purpose.

ACV Treatment

If you incur a cut, you should immediately clean the affected area with warm water and a chemical-free soap (soaps with added chemical ingredients can irritate cuts and abrasions). Then soak a gauze pad in a solution of one part ACV and one part water and apply the gauze over the cut, holding it in place with a bandage. This will help the cut to heal more quickly and also reduce the risk of scarring. Leave the bandage on overnight, and then replace with another ACV-soaked gauze bandage each day until your cut is fully healed.

What Else to Consider

Persistent cuts that do not heal and/or begin to present with pus should be cared for by a health professional.

DAMAGED AND DRY HAIR

See HAIR, DAMAGED AND DRY.

DANDRUFF

Dandruff is a common scalp condition in which dead skin on the scalp sheds, causing irritating white flakes that fall on the shoulders and clothes.

Symptoms

In some cases, dandruff can be accompanied by an itchy, scaly scalp, as well as greasy patches of skin.

Causes

The vast majority of dandruff cases are linked to a condition known as seborrheic dermatitis, a type of acidic, mild scalp inflammation accompanied by excessive secretions of oily fatty acids onto the scalp.

In addition to such fatty acid conditions, the other most cause of dandruff is bacteria growth on the scalp. Such bacteria can thrive on scalps that are overly acidic and oily. Other common causes of dandruff are commercial shampoos and related hair care products that contain irritating chemicals.

Benefits

Apple cider vinegar, applied topically to the scalp, can help minimize and possibly even eliminate dandruff problems. ACV acts as a dandruff remedy in a number of ways.

- First, it acts as a natural *astringent* and is effective for removing dead skin cells from the scalp.

- Second, it helps to balance scalp pH so that your scalp does not become too acidic. In fact, the pH of ACV is close to the natural pH of skin, so when ACV is applied to scalp it helps to maintain the the scalp's acid mantle. This, in turn, protects against foreign bacteria.

- Third, ACV helps cleanse the pores of the scalp, removing oils that may be clogging them.

- Finally, ACV helps to reduce scalp inflammation associated with dandruff while simultaneously improve circulation in the scalp, further helping to reduce dandruff.

ACV Treatment

To make a *topical dandruff solution* using apple cider vinegar, combine one-quarter to one-third cup of ACV with one cup of warm, pure, filtered water. Mix thoroughly, then apply to your scalp and hair, massaging the mixture into all areas of your scalp. Let the solution sit on the scalp for at least five minutes or until it dries, then rinse your scalp or hair with water and gently towel-dry your hair. You can apply the ACV *solution* twice a day, morning and evening. This solution also acts as a healthy, natural hair conditioner, rinse, and shampoo.

What Else to Consider

Since dandruff is most commonly caused by an overly acidic condition due to one's diet, if you continue to experience dandruff, consider consulting with a nutritionally-trained physician or certified clinical nutritionist who can help you create a healthier, more akalizing diet (also see the dietary recommendations in Chapter 5, beginning on page 43). To avoid bacterial overgrowth on your scalp, wash your scalp and hair regularly, and avoid the use of chemically-laden shampoos and other hair care products.

See also **HAIR, DAMAGED AND DRY.**

DIABETES (TYPE 2)

There are two types of diabetes, type 1 and type 2. In both cases, the conditions are associated with unhealthy, elevated blood glucose (blood sugar) levels.Type 2 diabetes is the most common type of diabetes, accounting for as much as 90 percent of all diabetes cases in the U.S. In cases of diabetes, while the pancreas remains capable of adequately producing enough insulin, due to a variety of factors the body becomes insulin-resistant, meaning even when enough insulin is being produced by the body, the insulin is unable to prevent excess blood sugar buildup.

Symptoms

By detecting the common symptoms of type 2 diabetes, you decrease the risk of developing the complications of diabetes. Early signs may include:

- Blurry vision
- Extreme and frequent thirst
- Extreme fatigue
- Feeling hungry though you are eating
- Frequent urination
- Slow healing cuts or bruises
- Tingling pain/numbness in hands or feet

Causes

In type 1 diabetes, blood glucose levels rise above healthy limits because they body is unable to produce enough insulin, which is vital for the proper metabolism of blood glucose, due to damage to the pancreas, the organ that primarily produces insulin. As a result, without the use of insulin drugs and other diabetes medications, sufferers of type 1 diabetes run the risk of blood glucose levels building up and the glucose spilling out into the urine. This results in cellular starvation because the body's cells are unable to obtain the necessary glucose they require to be properly nourished and to have enough energy to perform their many cellular functions. There is no known cure for type 1 diabetes, which requires daily insulin injections in order for sufferers of this condition to remain healthy and stay alive.

The primary factors that cause type 2 diabetes are poor diet (especially diets high in sugar and simple carbohydrates, excess levels of complex carbohydrates, junk foods, and soda and other sugary drinks), obesity, and a sedentary lifestyle. Despite the serious health threats type 2 diabetes poses, including increasing the risk of heart disease, stroke, and cancer, the incidence of type 2 diabetes in the U.S. continues to skyrocket and is projected to increase by at least 50 percent over the next two decades.

Benefits

Given the scientific studies that confirm apple cider vinegar's ability to help regulate blood sugar levels (*see* page 87), it should not be surprising to learn that ACV offers benefit for type 2 diabetes, as well. This fact has been verified in both animal and human studies. A number of these studies have been published in *Diabetes Care,* the official, peer-reviewed medical journal of the American Diabetes Association.

One of the most significant of these studies was conducted in 2004 by Carol S. Johnston, Ph.D, R.D., Professor and Associate Director of the Nutrition Program in the School of Nutrition and Health Promotion at Arizona State University, and two of her colleagues. In that study, a total of 29 participants were tested. The participants were divided into three groups. Eight of the participants where healthy, 11 of them were insulin-resistant and at risk for developing type 2 diabetes, and 10 of the participants had been diagnosed with type 2 diabetes. None of the study participants were taking diabetes medications when the study was conducted.

In all three groups, the test subjects were randomly assigned to consume either a vinegar drink consisting of 20 grams (approximately 0.7 ounces) of apple cider vinegar, approximately one and a half ounces of water, and 1 teaspoon of saccharine or a placebo drink. Two minutes later, all subjects ate a high carbohydrate test meal consisting of a white bagel, butter, and orange juice. In total, the meal was made up of 87 grams of total carbohydrates.

Prior to the study, all participants had sample of their blood collected and analyzed to determine their fasting and post-meal glucose and insulin levels. At the end of one week, additional blood samples were collected at fasting and 30 and 60 minutes after the same meal and the subjects' glucose and insulin levels were reexamined. The study revealed that all three subject groups have better glucose and insulin readings when they consumed the ACV drink before their meals compared to when they consumed the placebo drink. Most significantly, the people in the pre-diabetes group benefited the most from consuming their ACV drink, experiencing an average reduction of their blood glucose levels of nearly 50 percent. They also exhibited lower blood glucose levels than the healthy participants after both groups consumed the ACV drink. The diabetic group also showed significant benefit from consuming the ACV drink, exhibiting an average 25 percent reduction in their blood glucose levels.

In a subsequent long-term study conducted by Dr. Johnston and her colleagues and published in 2013, 14 test subjects with a clinically observed high risk for developing type 2 diabetes, including eight participants who were already pre-diabetic, were tested during a 12-week period. As with the previous study, none of the test subjects were using diabetes medications. The study participants were divided into two groups, seven of whom served as the control group, and seven of whom either consumed two tablespoons of apple cider vinegar or ACV pills prior to lunch and dinner for the entire 12-week period. Both groups had their blood glucose levels analyzed prior to the study, and their glucose levels were measured again twice each day, once upon waking in a fasting state, and once 2 hours after a meal. All of the participants followed their usual dietary habits and maintained their normal levels of physical activity throughout the testing period.

The study showed an immediate and sustained reduction in the fasting glucose levels of the participants who consumed the two tablespoons of ACV compared to the control group and the group who took the ACV pills (one more reason why liquid ACV is superior to ACV capsules and pills; for more on why you should avoid ACV capsules and pills, *see* Chapter 3, page 31). In the group who took liquid ACV, the reduction of their fasting glucose levels were nearly 400 percent greater than for the group who took ACV pills. Both the groups who took ACV as either a liquid or in pill form also showed significant reductions in their blood glucose levels 2 hours after their meals. As a result of this study, Dr. Johnston wrote, "These results support a therapeutic effect for [apple cider] vinegar in individuals at risk for T2D [type 2 diabetes], including those diagnosed with prediabetes."

In 2007 study, Dr. Johnston and her colleague Andrea M. White, PhD, also found that that ingesting two tablespoons of apple cider vinegar before bedtime lowered the morning blood glucose levels of four men and seven women, all of whom had previously been diagnosed with type 2 diagnosis. This reduction was double that experienced by a control group, with an average reduction of between four and six percent. Moreover, the greatest reductions occurred in participants who, prior to the beginning of the test, were shown to have the highest fasting blood glucose levels.

ACV Treatment

Based on the above studies, if you are pre-diabetic or have been diagnosed with type 2 diabetes, you can follow approaches similar to those in the studies above. Rather than consuming two tablespoons undiluted apple cider vinegar, however, I recommend combining that amount of ACV with eight ounces of pure, filtered water and drinking a glass before each meal.

What Else to Consider

Type 2 diabetes is a chronic degenerative disease. If you suffer from it, or if you are pre-diabetic, seek the help of a physician or other health practitioner skilled in effectively treating both conditions. Unlike type 1 diabetes, type 2 diabetes, and especially pre-diabetes, can be completely reversed by following a healthy, low-carbohydrate diet, avoiding sugars and other sugary foods and drinks, and adopting a proper exercise program. Losing weight, if necessary, is also vitally important. Both type 2 diabetes and pre-diabetes are in the vast majority of cases the result of ongoing, unhealthy lifestyle choices. When such choices are eliminated, you may be surprised by how quickly type 2 diabetes can be completely reversed. I personally know doctors who routinely eliminate their patients' type 2 diabetes and pre-diabetic conditions in as little as one to three months, including in patients who previously needed to use diabetes medications for years, primarily through dietary and nutritional interventions, along with appropriate exercise and weight loss programs.

DIAPER RASH

Diaper rash is a very common ailment that affects young infants. It typically appears on the skin under a diaper in children younger than 2 years old however, it can also be noticed in incontinent adults.

Symptoms

Your baby's diaper rash can be identified by an area pink or red in color with raised bumps in the buttocks, thighs, or genitals. The bumps may contain fluid.

Causes

It is caused by moisture due to wet or soiled diapers, causing irritation on the baby's backside which can be compounded by bacteria growth for which the moisture from the diapers acts as a breeding ground. New foods introduced into your baby's diet may also cause a diaper rash.

Benefits

A gentle wash with an apple cider vinegar solution can help relieve the discomfort of diaper rash. More importantly, ACV can also help repair the affect skin area because it acts as a natural *astringent* and is effective for removing dead skin cells. ACV also helps to balance skin pH so that the baby's affected backside does not become too acidic. In fact, the pH of ACV is close to the natural pH of skin, so when ACV is applied to skin it helps to maintain the skin's acid mantle. This, in turn, protects against bacteria. Finally, ACV helps to reduce skin inflammation while simultaneously improving circulation in the skin, further helping diaper rash to heal.

ACV Treatment

To make a *topical solution* using apple cider vinegar, combine one-quarter to one-third cup of ACV with one cup of lukewarm, pure, filtered water. Then soak a small cotton towel (you can also use a cotton swab) in the solution and gently cleanse the baby's backside. Repeat every hour or so until the diaper rash heals.

What Else to Consider

To prevent diaper rash, change wet or soiled diapers promptly and be sure to cleanse your baby's backside thoroughly before applying new diapers. Also do not apply diapers until your baby's backside is completely dry. In addition, avoid washing your baby with chemically-laden soaps. Instead of bath wipes, which can also irritate infant skin, wash your baby's backside with water and a cotton wash cloth or cotton balls. Persistent diaper rash may be a sign of skin infection. If it persists, consult your pediatrician.

DIARRHEA

Diarrhea is not a health condition, per se, but rather a symptom of and means by which your body responds to other illnesses. Occasional bouts of diarrhea (loose, watery, and more frequent bowel movements) are quite common. However, diarrhea that persists for more than a few days requires medical attention due to the increased risk of dehydration and nutrient loss that persistent diarrhea has.

Symptoms

Symptoms characterized by diarrhea may include:

- Abdominal cramps and pain
- Bloating
- Blood in stools
- Nausea
- Watery, loose bowel movement

Causes

Diarrhea can be caused by a number of diseases and conditions, such as food poisoning, infection, viruses, parasites, medications, and digestive disorders.

Food allergies, especially to milk and other dairy products that contain lactose, can also cause diarrhea, as can eating junk food (due to the chemicals they contain) and drinking contaminated water.

During bouts of diarrhea, it is very important that you keep your body hydrated by drinking lots of pure, filtered water until your symptoms subside. During the early stages of diarrhea it is also a good idea to not eat, aside from fruits. Bananas are especially good during this time because of their potassium content. Potassium acts as an electrolyte in the body, and electrolytes can be rapidly lost during bouts of diarrhea. (Electrolytes regulate the electric charge on your body's cells and the flow of water across their membranes and also carry electrical impulses from the nerves that control your body's tissue function and movement.)

As diarrhea symptoms begin to ease, you can add nutritious soups and steamed vegetables, returning to a normal, healthy diet once your symptoms have fully subsided. It may also be a good idea to supplement with a multivitamin/mineral product to help your body better cope with the loss of nutrients that diarrhea can cause. Avoid taking high doses of vitamin C, however, as this can cause or prolong diarrhea symptoms.

Benefit

Apple cider vinegar can often help speed up recovery from diarrhea. It does so because of its ability to fight off infection, especially infections related to food poisoning. In addition, ACV contains pectin, a natural fiber that helps prevent and relieve diarrhea, as well enzymes and nutrients such as potassium that are also helpful for healing diarrhea. ACV also acts as a natural prebiotic, meaning it helps the body replenish its own supply of healthy intestinal flora, further aiding the body as it copes with diarrhea symptoms.

ACV Treatment

One of the best ways to use ACV to treat diarrhea is to make an ACV *tonic* (one to two tablespoons of ACV added to eight ounces of pure, filtered water). Instead of drinking it all at once, however, sip it slowly over the course of 10 to 15 minutes. You can then repeat this process every 1 to 2 hours until your diarrhea subsides.

What Else to Consider

If your diarrhea persists, see a doctor. You should also see a doctor if you suffer from regular bouts of diarrhea, even if they are not long in duration. Frequent diarrhea can be a sign of food allergies, nutritional and/or enzyme deficiencies, or chronic infections within the gastrointestinal tract. Parasite infections, which are far more common than most people, including doctors, realize, may also be a contributing factors. A physician trained in detecting and addressing such factors can be very valuable in helping you resolve your diarrhea symptoms.

See also **FOOD POISONING and INFECTION.**

EARACHE

Earaches can occur at any time during the course of one's lifetime, yet it most commonly occurs in young children. The pain, which may be dull or a sharp sensation, may be constant or it may come and go.

Symptoms

Besides ear pain, symptoms of an ear infection may include:

- Balance problems
- Difficulty sleeping
- Feeling irritable
- Fever
- Loss of appetite
- Pulling at an ear

Causes

An earache is usually caused by the buildup of fluid or inflammation in the middle ear. Such buildups can cause pressure that swells and closes the ear's eustachian tube. When this tube narrows because of swelling, fluid from the middle ear becomes obstructed, accumulates, and can turn stagnant causing acute ear pain and also serving as a breeding ground for bacterial infections.

Benefit

Earaches can sometimes respond to eardrops of apple cider vinegar and water. This is due to ACV's antibacterial and antiseptic properties.

ACV Treatment

To make ACV *eardrops* mix equal portions of ACV and warm, pure filtered water. Mix thoroughly, then fill up an eyedropper with the solution. Slowly apply drops of the solution into the ear, wait for 30 seconds, then tilt the ear downward so that the solution seeps out, clearing the ear. You can repeat this process a few times a day until the condition subsides.

Do **NOT** overdo the amount of ACV *eardrop solution* you apply to the ear, and never apply ACV alone. Also be aware that the use of ACV *eardrops* can sometimes cause fleeting symptoms of vertigo, since our ears are responsible for helping us maintain our balance. If this happens, the sensations should pass quickly, but you should not continue using the ACV *eardrop solution.* Also always consult with a pediatrician first before using any self-care remedy on children.

What Else to Consider

Poor, diet, nutritional deficiencies, bacterial infections, and the overuse of antibiotics can all cause or contribute to earache. To most effectively prevent and treat earache it is essential that its underlying causes be determined and addressed, something that is best done with the help of a holistically-trained, integrative pediatrician (for earache in infants and children) or physician. Keeping the ears properly cleaned and free of buildup is also important.

ECZEMA

Eczema, also known as dermatitis, is a skin condition characterized by inflammation. There are various types of eczema that are based on where and how they manifest on the body.

Symptoms

Eczema is usually accompanied by one or more of the following symptoms:

- Blisters
- Itching
- Rash
- Reddish bumps
- Scaly skin, and/or crusting of the skin

In some cases, the affected skin area may also ooze pus. Eczema can occur anywhere on the body.

Causes

Essentially all cases of eczema are caused by one or more of the following factors:

- Chemical exposures
- Food and/or environmental allergies
- Low stomach acid (hydrochloric acid, or HCl)
- Nutritional deficiencies
- Poor diet

Excessive secretions of oily fatty acids onto the skin can also cause or exacerbate eczema due to bacterial overgrowth that such acids can trigger. Bacteria thrive on skin that is overly acidic and oily.

Treatment of eczema should be overseen by a dermatologist. Working with a physician with a background in nutritional medicine and allergies can also be helpful. Other common causes of scalp problems are commercial shampoos and related hair care products that contain irritating chemicals, all of which should be avoided.

Benefits

Apple cider vinegar applied topically to the skin can help minimize and eliminate eczema problems. ACV acts as an eczema remedy in a number of ways.

- First, it acts as a natural *astringent* and is effective for removing dead skin cells from the skin.

- Second, it helps to balance skin pH so that your skin does not become too acidic. In fact, the pH of ACV is close to the natural pH of skin, so when ACV is applied to skin it helps to maintain the skin's acid mantle. This, in turn, protects against foreign bacteria.

- Third, ACV helps cleanse the pores of the skin, removing oils that may be clogging them.

- Finally, ACV helps to reduce scalp inflammation while simultaneously improve circulation in the skin.

ACV Treatment

To make a *topical scalp solution* using apple cider vinegar, combine one-quarter to one-third cup of ACV with one cup of warm, pure, filtered water. Mix thoroughly, then soak a clean, cotton wash cloth or towel in the mixture. Apply the cloth or towel to the affected, holding it in place for 20 to 30 minutes. Repeat as necessary, or least once a day (morning and evenings).

Drinking one or more glasses of apple cider vinegar *tonic* can also sometimes help heal eczema because of its acetic acid content, which can help improve stomach acid levels. As we age, the amount of hydrochloric acid produced by our stomachs usually declines. Apple cider vinegar supplies added acid to the stomach, helping cases of eczema where HCl deficiencies are a causative factor. If you suffer from eczema, combine one or two tablespoons of ACV to one eight-ounce glass of pure, filtered water, and drink it 20 minutes before each meal. Try to do this before every meal.

What Else to Consider

Since eczema problems can be caused or made worse by an overly acidic condition due to one's diet, if you continue to experience eczema problems consider consulting with a nutritionally-trained physician or certified clinical nutritionist who can help your create a healthier, more akalizing diet (also see the dietary recommendations in Chapter 5, beginning on page 43). To avoid bacterial overgrowth on your skin, bathe or shower regularly, wear clean clothes, and avoid the use of chemically-laden soaps and other body cleansing and hair care products.

See also ALLERGIES, INFLAMMATION, NUTRIENT ABSORPTION AND NUTRITIONAL DEFICIENCIES, RASHES, and SKIN CONDITIONS.

FATIGUE

All of us experience fatigue from time to time, and for many of us fatigue can be a common everyday experience. So much so that many people cannot function properly in the morning without first reaching for one or two cups of coffee or some other caffeinated drink. While a few cups of coffee each day has been shown to provide a number of health benefits, excess consumption of coffee and other caffeine beverages can compromise health, including impairing adrenal gland function and causing chronic, low-grade dehydration.

Symptoms

Fatigue is a symptom triggered by an underlying disease or condition. It is characterized by feeling weak to being constantly tired or lacking energy.

Causes

There are a number of causes of fatigue ranging from those conditions that cause a poor blood supply to diseases that affect metabolism, as well as infections, viruses, and disorders that trigger sleep disturbances.

Benefit

ACV contains potassium and other electrolytes, both of which are necessary for proper energy production. (Electrolytes regulate the electric charge on your body's cells and the flow of water across their membranes and also carry electrical impulses from the nerves that control your body's tissue function and movement.) The B vitamins that ACV contains are also necessary for proper energy production by your body. Moreover, ACV acts as a natural antioxidant and can help protect against free-radical damage that can cause energy loss and premature aging of your body's cell, tissues, and organs.

ACV Treatment

A glass of apple cider vinegar in water (one to two tablespoons of ACV added to eight ounces of pure, filtered water) can provide a healthy alternative to caffeine drinks while also helping to banish fatigue. ACV's energizing properties are due to a number of reasons (*see* page 119).

To further improve your energy levels, you can also try drinking a glass or two of switchel each day. As you learned in Chapter 1, switchel drinks were widely used by American farmers beginning in the 18th century to help keep them energized as they worked long days planting, growing and harvesting their crops, tending to their animals, and harvesting and baling hay during hay season. To make switchel drinks at home, simply add a tablespoon of raw, organic honey to your ACV *tonic*. You can find other switchel recipes in Chapter 4 (*see* page 41).

What Else to Consider

To improve your resistance to fatigue, be sure to eat a healthy diet, stay properly hydrated, get regular exercise, manage your stress levels, and get enough sleep each night. For more on how to do so, see the recommendations I shared with you in Chapter 5.

While feelings of fatigue are increasingly common today, persistent fatigue should not be ignored, as it is often a sign of more serious underlying conditions, which can range from chronic infections, nutrient deficiencies, and hormone imbalances, to liver disease and cancer. If you suffer from chronic fatigue, seek immediate medical attention.

FLATULENCE

Flatulence, or the passing of gas, is a natural occurrence that is caused by the buildup of intestinal gas (flatus) that is formed by the fermentation of food, especially carbohydrates. Often the food is not properly digested. In some cases, however, gas buildup in the intestines can cause distention of the abdomen and/or abdominal pains.

Symptoms

Normally, aside from the need to expel gas, flatulence does not present with any other symptoms.

Causes

The primary causes of flatulence are poor diet, a diet high in carbohydrate foods, food allergies, overeating, eating quickly, nutritional deficiencies, and lack of enzymes. Various gastrointestinal problems can also cause flatulence.

To minimize the occurrence of flatulence avoid overeating, chew your food slowly and thoroughly before swallowing, and eat more high fiber foods. Taking digestive enzymes at the start of each meal can also help reduce the incidence of flatulence.

Benefits

The acetic acid in ACV helps maintain healthy levels of stomach acids, which are necessary for the proper digestion of the foods you eat. ACV also contains enzymes, further aiding the complete digestion of foods.

ACV Treatment

A glass of apple cider vinegar *tonic* (one to two tablespoons of ACV added to eight ounces of pure, filtered water) consumed before each meal can also help reduce flatulence.

What Else to Consider

Frequent flatulence is not normal and may be a sign of more serious underlying health conditions, food allergies, and/or nutritional deficiencies. If you experience frequent bouts of flatulence, don't ignore them. Check with your doctor to determine what factors may be involved so that they can be properly addressed.

See also **NUTRITIONAL DEFICIENCIES and GASTROINTESTINAL PROBLEMS.**

FOOD POISONING

Food poisoning refers to any gastrointestinal problem that occurs as a result of eating contaminated food or drinking contaminated beverages. Although most cases of food poisoning occur within 30 minutes to 1 or 2 hours after such foods or beverages are consumed, in some cases symptoms may not present until 48 hours or more after the offending foods or drinks are consumed.

Symptoms

Symptoms of food poisoning vary. The most common symptoms are diarrhea, vomiting, abdominal cramping, fever, sweating, dehydration, and fatigue.

Causes

The most common food contaminants are E. coli and salmonella, but any food-borne pathogen, both bacterial and viral can cause food poisoning.

Benefits

To speed recovery of food poisoning it is important to get proper rest and to keep yourself hydrated by drinking plenty of pure, filtered water.

Apple cider vinegar can be effective in helping to counteract food poisoning for a number of reasons. First, it contains potassium and other electrolytes, both of which are necessary for proper energy production, and which can be quickly depleted by food poisoning, especially when diarrhea is involved. (Electrolytes regulate the electric charge on your body's cells and the flow of water across their membranes and also carry electrical impulses from the nerves that control your body's tissue function and movement.) ACV also contains pectin, which acts as a natural fiber that can help move contaminated food waste products in the intestines out of the body. The acetic acid and other acid compounds ACV contains can also help because of how they act as natural prebiotics, helping to stimulate the growth of healthy bacteria in the GI tract that can help neutralize food-borne pathogens. These compounds also act as natural enzymes, further aiding in the recovery from food poisoning.

ACV's antibacterial and antiviral properties also help to prevent and reduce bacterial and viral infections in the stomach and the rest of the GI tract. This is particularly true of the acetic acid in ACV, which has been proven to be highly effective for neutralizing both E. coli and salmonella.

ACV Treatment

Organic herbal teas, such as chamomile or peppermint tea, can also be helpful, as can apple cider vinegar *tonic* drinks (one to two tablespoons of ACV added to eight ounces of pure, filtered water). If you suffer from food poisoning, make a glass of ACV *tonic* and sip it slowly over the course of 10 to 15 minutes. Repeat every 1 to 2 hours until your symptoms subside.

Finally, a glass of ACV *tonic* before meals can help improve the level of stomach acids. Proper stomach acid levels are essential both for healthy digestion, but also for preventing infections in the stomach and the rest of the GI tract.

What Else to Consider

If your symptoms of food poisoning are severe, seek immediate medical attention, especially if severe diarrhea and/or vomiting occur. If available, also bring samples of the suspect foods or drinks so that they can be tested. In all cases of food poisoning, you should avoid eating any solid foods until your symptoms pass, while continuing to drink plenty of pure, filtered water and/or organic, herbal teas.

To avoid food poisoning, minimize how often you dine out, or only eat at restaurants you are familiar with and trust. When traveling, only drink bottled water and avoid salads and uncooked vegetables, as these can often be kept on ice made from contaminated water. Taking digestive enzymes before your meals can also help, as can charcoal tablets after meals.

See also **DIARRHEA and FATIGUE.**

FOOT ODOR

Bromodosis or foot odor can affect anyone. Foot odor is a common year-round foot skin issue. It can be uncomfortable as well as embarrassing.

Symptoms

Foot odor symptoms are not difficult to recognize. The most common indications are sweaty, smelly feet or smelly shoes.

Causes

Foot odor, like body odor in general, is most commonly caused by dried sweat on the skin for a few hours. During this time, skin bacteria decompose the sweat, causing feet to smell. Foot odor is most often the result of feet being kept in socks and shoes or other footwear that creates an airless, warm environment that is ideal for sweat buildup. It can also be the result of foot or toenail fungus.

Benefits

Like other types of body odor, foot odor can be prevented or at least significantly minimized by healthy hygiene practices, including showering or bathing on a daily basis.

Just as apple cider vinegar offers a safe, effective, and very inexpensive alternative to store-bought deodorants and antiperspirants, so too can ACV help mitigate food odor through the use of an ACV foot soak.

ACV Treatment

Simply add equal parts of ACV and comfortably hot water together in a pan or pail large enough to fit both of your feet in comfortably. Mix the ACV and water thoroughly, then soak your feet for 20 to 30 minutes. If foot or toenail fungus is involved, you can omit the water and simply do a *foot soak* with ACV.

What Else to Consider

If your foot odor persists consult with your doctor or a podiatrist to determine what underlying causes may be contributing to your problem. Also be sure to follow proper hygiene, including taking a daily shower or bath, and wearing clean socks, changing them daily, and clean, comfortable footwear.

See also **FOOT AND TOENAIL FUNGUS.**

FOOT AND TOENAIL FUNGUS

Both foot and toenail fungus are rather common, unsightly conditions. Foot fungus is more commonly known as athlete's foot, while toenail fungus is known as *onychomycosis*. Both foot and toenail fungus feed on keratin, a type of protein nutrient found in the cells of our skin and nails. When fungus comes in contact with keratin it quickly begins to break it down, causing the skin of the feet and toes to become scaly and flaky and toenails to become discolored and brittle.

Symptoms

Symptoms of foot and toenail fungus vary. Fungus on the skin of the feet or toes include reddish, cracked skin, skin peeling, itching, burning and stinging sensations, blistering and, sometimes, bleeding. When fungus is located on the toenail itself it can cause toenail to become discolored (usually turning yellow or brown) and abnormally thick. White markings can sometimes appear on the nail, as well. Both foot and toenail fungus can result in a foul odor.

Causes

Both foot and toenail fungus is caused by a class of fungi called *dermatophytes*, which are related to yeasts and molds. Although foot and toenail fungus is rare among children, the risks for developing them increases significantly as we age. Approximately 50 percent of all Americans will develop one or both conditions at least once before age 70.

Dermatophytes and other types of fungus thrive in warm, moist places, such as public showers, locker rooms, swimming pools, and even personal showers that are shared by family members. Once the fungus takes hold, it can be highly contagious (which is why so many people contract athlete's foot when using public showers).

Benefits

Both foot and toenail fungus should be treated as early as possible. The longer that you wait for treatment, the more difficult the fungus may become to treat. Medical treatment options vary, depending on the severity and location (skin or nail) of the infection, and include prescription, antifungal drugs (both oral and topical), antifungal powders, medicated toenail polish, and medical laser treatments.

Apple cider vinegar can often enhance the effectiveness of such treatments, both when consumed as an ACV tonic or applied topically. ACV's benefits for treating foot and toenail fungus derive from the acetic acid and natural enzymes it contains, all of which can help neutralize fungus growth on the feet and toenails.

ACV Treatment

To augment an overall foot or toenail fungus treatment plan, drink three glasses of apple cider vinegar *tonic* each day. For each glass, add one tablespoon of ACV to eight ounces of pure, filtered water. Or you can try filling a water bottle with ACV and water and sip it throughout the day.

You can apply apple cider vinegar *topically* over the affected areas. Unless you have sensitive skin, there is no need to dilute the ACV. You can also *soak* your feet in an ACV foot bath. Simply add three to four cups of ACV to a comfortable, hot foot bath and soak for 20 to 30 minutes once a day.

What Else to Consider

As mentioned, to properly treat foot and toenail fungus infections, you need to seek the immediate help a podiatrist or other health professional who knows how to most effectively deal with it. In addition, you need to be sure to properly clean your feet and toes every day. You should also avoid sharing towels or nail clippers with anyone else, and avoid walking barefoot in wet, public places (gyms, locker rooms, and public pools and showers). Also, if possible, wear shoes made of breathable materials (natural, absorbent fibers) and in warm weather, when going outside, wear sandals. In addition, change your socks every day, and when inside your home go barefoot.

See also **FOOT ODOR.**

GALLBLADDER PROBLEMS

Your gallbladder, which is located beneath your liver, is responsible for delivering bile, which it receives and stores from the liver, into the intestines following a meal. The bile is then used to breakdown fats contained in food. Like your liver, your gallbladder is also an organ of detoxification, as the bile it secretes also helps to eliminate toxins and waste matter.

Symptoms

Recognizing the following symptoms will help you deal with a gallbladder problem:

- Abdominal pain, tenderness on right side
- Bloating
- Changes in stool color and consistency
- Chest pain
- Discolored urine
- Fever
- Frequency of urination
- Indigestion
- Loss of appetite
- Nausea
- Vomiting

Causes

Disorders of the gallbladder are mostly caused by gall stones. Risk factors that may contribute to the development of gallstones is a diet high in fat and cholesterol, being overweight, age, and family history.

Benefits

Just as apple cider vinegar can assist liver function, so too can it help to keep your gallbladder healthy and prevent the formation of gallstones, which are formed from a combination of bile and cholesterol and other compounds, and can cause various complications, including blocking the bile duct and causing the gallbladder to become inflamed. When this happens, surgery to remove the gallbladder may be required.

The cholesterol-lowering effects of apple cider vinegar, acetic acid, its main component, and polyphenols, which ACV also contains, have been proven by scientific research. By keeping cholesterol levels in check, ACV can help minimize the risk of gallstone formation.

ACV Treatment

Drinking one or more glasses of ACV *tonic* each day (one to two tablespoons

ACV added to eight ounces of pure, filtered water) can help prevent gallstone formation and help keep your gallbladder healthy.

See also **CHOLESTEROL, LIVER FUNCTION and TOXIC OVERLOAD.**

GASTROINTESTINAL PROBLEMS

Just as apple cider vinegar can help prevent and reverse constipation, diarrhea, flatulence, and food poisoning, ACV can also be helpful for relieving various other gastrointestinal problems, such as indigestion, mild stomachache, and minor cases of GI tract pain.

Symptoms

Symptoms of gastrointestinal disorders may include:

- Constipation
- Diarrhea
- Gassy or bloated feeling
- GI bleeding
- Nausea
- Stomach pain
- Vomiting

Causes

Gastrointestinal problems are generally caused by a lack of digestive enzymes, lack of stomach acid, and/or bacterial overgrowth in the GI tract, as well as by a variety of factors, including:

- Chronic low-grade dehydration
- Chronic stress
- Emotional upsets
- Food allergies
- Impaired nutrition
- Lack of exercise
- Poor diet
- Use of pharmaceutical drugs (over time can cause constipation and other GI imbalances)

Benefits

To avoid or reverse gastrointestinal problems it is important to follow a diet of healthy, nutritious, fiber-rich foods, keep your body adequately hydrated, engage in regular exercise, and avoid eating meals when you are stressed or emotionally upset. Sugar, simple carbohydrates, fried foods, caffeine, and alcohol can also cause or contribute to GI problems, and therefore should also be avoided.

Apple cider vinegar can also help prevent and relieve GI symptoms.

ACV is able to do this for a variety of reasons, including because of its pectin content (pectin acts as a natural fiber). The acetic acid and other acid compounds ACV contains can also help resolve mild GI problems in the following ways:

- First, they act as natural prebiotics, helping stimulate the growth of healthy bacteria in the GI tract that aid digestion and help to keep us regular.

- Second, these compounds in ACV also act as natural enzymes, further aiding digestion.

- Third, ACV's antibacterial and antiviral properties help to prevent and reduce bacterial and viral infections in the stomach and the GI tract.

- Finally, a glass of ACV tonic before meals improves the level of stomach acids. Proper stomach acid levels are essential both for healthy digestion, preventing infections in the stomach and the rest of the GI tract.

ACV Treatment

If you suffer from mild gastrointestinal problems, try drinking one to three glasses of apple cider vinegar *tonic* each day (one tablespoon of ACV combined with eight ounces of pure, filtered water), ideally 20 minutes before each meal.

What Else to Consider

Chronic gastrointestinal problems, no matter how minor they may seem, should not be ignored. If you suffer from such problems on an ongoing basis, seek prompt medical attention.

See also CONSTIPATION, DIARRHEA, FLATULENCE, and FOOD POISONING.

GINGIVITIS

Gingivitis is a form of gum disease caused by infectious bacteria that can accumulate in plaque and under the teeth and within the gum lining.

Symptoms

Symptoms of gingivitis include swelling and inflammation of the gums, as well as bleeding of the gums, especially during flossing and when teeth are brushed. Early stage gingivitis is usually harmless. Left untreated, however, it can lead to periodontitis, a much more serious type of gum disease that can cause teeth to loosen from the gums and jawbone, as well as pocketing within the gums, and even deterioration of the jawbone. In addition, as bacteria in plaque and beneath the gum line builds up some of the bacteria and the toxins they produce can migrate past the mouth, into the throat, and then move on into the bloodstream, causing the body's immune system to become suppressed. In recent years, scientists have discovered that such bacteria can increase the risk of chronic, unhealthy inflammation in the body, and even contribute to heart disease and stroke. Therefore, the best course of action is to treat and resolve gingivitis before it can progress further.

Causes

The primary cause of gingivitis is plaque buildup and poor dental hygiene. But other factors can also be involved, including poor dietary habits, nutritional deficiencies, and unhealthy lifestyle habits such as smoking. In women, the hormonal fluctuations that can occur during pregnancy, menstruation, and menopause can also contribute to gingivitis because such fluctuations can make gums become more sensitive and therefore more susceptible to bacterial infections.

Benefits

To help prevent gingivitis, it is important that you follow proper dental hygiene, including regular brushing of your teeth and flossing of your gums. Gargling with a mouthwash can also be helpful. Unfortunately, most commercial mouthwashes contain a variety of ingredients that aren't safe if swallowed. Apple cider vinegar in the form of a gargle or mouth rinse offers a safe and effective alternative.

ACV is helpful for preventing gingivitis for the same reasons that it can help prevent bad breath. ACV's antibacterial and antiseptic properties make it an ideal natural solution for treating bacteria on your teeth, gums, and tongue.

ACV Treatment

Making an apple cider vinegar *mouthwash* or *rinse* is very easy. Simply combine on tablespoon of ACV with half a cup of pure, filtered water. Mix thoroughly, then swish or gargle in your mouth for 30 to 60 seconds, then spit the mixture out. Repeat as necessary. For best results, do this after you first brush your teeth and floss your gums in the morning and before going to bed.

Do not swish or gargle with apple cider vinegar that is not diluted in water. Because of its acidic content undiluted ACV can potentially harm the enamel of your teeth.

What Else to Consider

If you suffer from chronic gingivitis, please see your dentist, so that you can be sure of doing all that you need to do to prevent gingivitis from progressing further. Ideally, you should see your dentist every six months or at least once a year so that he or she can monitor your overall dental health.

See also **BAD BREATH.**

HAIR, DAMAGED AND DRY

Having healthy, beautiful hair is a high priority for most people, and high on the list of what they are willing to pay for. All across the globe people, especially women, spend a fortune on hair care products. According to an analysis by the Wall Street firm Goldman Sachs, in 2003 the annual global expenditure on hair care products is about $38 billion. By 2015, that number had risen to $100 billion in the United States alone which is twice as much as Americans spend on dental care. And according to *The Economist*, Americans also spend more each year on hair care and other beauty products than they do on education.

Symptoms

While the shampoos, conditioners, hair rinses, and other hair care products can certainly give the appearance of healthy hair, in reality many commercial hair care products are not healthy for you, containing, as they do, a variety of chemicals and abrasives. Not only can such ingredients damage hair when used regularly, they can also cause other health problems. Some of them can also be carcinogenic, meaning they can cause cancer. Cancer-causing ingredients found in many hair care products include substances such as phthalates, parabens, sodium lauryl sulfate, and even coal tar. Given that fact, hair care products containing such ingredients should be avoided.

Another reason why most commercial hair care products should be avoided is because they have an alkaline pH that is harmful to hair's cuticle "seal." The cuticle seal is the outermost part of the hair shaft. It gives hair its strength and is responsible for protecting the cortex of the hair shaft. The hair cortex is the thickest layer of hair and contains most of the hair's pigment, called melanin. Melanin is what gives hair its color. Alkaline hair care products harm the hair cuticle seal, causing it to open, which can cause hair to weaken, break, and become dry, limp, and dull in appearance.

Benefits

Fortunately, apple cider vinegar offers a safe, very inexpensive, and very effective alternative to commercial hair care products, making it an ideal for use as a combination shampoo, conditioner, and hair rinse. ACV's hair restorative properties are due in part to its pH, which is close to the pH of the hair and scalp. This not only enables ACV to maintain the health of the hair cuticle seal and keep it closed, but to also store shine and body to hair that has become dull, limp, and frizzy. ACV can also help prevent and repair hair split ends.

In addition, ACV when applied to hair and the scalp can help to prevent and eliminate dandruff and prevent the bacterial overgrowth that is often a factor in other scalp conditions. Due to its *astringent* qualities, ACV can also remove excess oils, dirt and other debris in both the hair and scalp. By doing so, ACV can help restore hair's natural shine and give it more bounce.

ACV Treatment

You can easily make your own all-in-one hair shampoo, conditioner and rinse at home. To do so, combine one-quarter cup of ACV with one cup of pure, filtered water. Mix thoroughly, then pour the mixture into a clean, empty squirt bottle. Then spray your hair and scalp with the mixture, gently massaging it into all areas of your hair and scalp just as you would do when using regular shampoo. When you finish, let the mixture remain in your hair and scalp for five minutes, then gently rinse it off using slightly warm water. To further condition your hair, before rinsing, you can let the mixture sit on your hair and scalp for 20 to 30 minutes, covering your hair with a shower cap once you are done massaging the ACV *mixture* into your scalp and hair. Then gently rinse in warm water. When drying your hair, gently towel dry rather than using a hair blower.

What Else to Consider

Keeping your hair and scalp clean is not only important for your overall appearance but also for your overall health. If you continue to experience unhealthy hair or scalp problems, consult with a holistically oriented hairdresser, stylist, cosmetician, or dermatologist.

See also DANDRUFF and SCALP PROBLEMS.

HEADACHE

Headache is a common health condition that can be minor or serious, depending on the type of headache it is and what is causing it.

Symptoms

The most common headache symptoms linked with the various types of headaches include:

- Aching head
- Dull pain
- Tenderness (scalp, neck, and should muscles)

- Tightness or pressure (forehead, sides, and back of head)

Causes

There are over ten primary types of headache categories, ranging from common tension headache to migraine headache, cluster headache, and headaches caused by physical trauma, sinus headache, headache caused by eyestrain, headache due to musculo-skeletal misalignments and other problems, and vascular headache, among others. Headache can also be caused by food allergies, nutritional deficiencies, chronic, low-grade dehydration, toxins, eyestrain, stress, and dental factors, such as temporomandibular joint (TMJ) syndrome. Persistent headache can also be a symptom of more serious health conditions, including brain tumors.

Benefits

While apple cider vinegar by itself is not a cure for any type of headache, most especially those that are structural in nature or related to vascular issues, eyestrain, of TMJ, ACV can help relieve headaches that are triggered by nutritional deficiencies, dehydration, toxicity, or sinus issues, and in some cases headache related to food allergies.

ACV's benefits for these types of headaches are due to the overall nutrient, enzyme, and acid compounds it contains. Working synergistically together, these ingredients in ACV help to restore nutritional deficiencies, relieve dehydration, and eliminate toxins in the body. ACV can also help improve circulation in the body, which, in turn, can help alleviate muscle tension in the body that may be contributing to headache.

ACV Treatment

If you suffer from any of the types of headache for which ACV may be helpful, try drinking one or more glasses of apple cider vinegar *tonic* (one to tablespoons of ACV added to eight ounces of pure, filter water) once or more each day until your headache symptoms fade away.

What Else to Consider

If you suffer from recurring or persistent headache you should seek medical attention to rule out or address any underlying health conditions that may be causing them. Also be sure to keep yourself properly hydrated, follow a healthy diet, get enough sleep, regular, but not excessive exercise, and do your best to manage stress. A soothing hot bath and/or a massage can also be helpful for relieving muscle tension that can contribute to headache, as can yoga, meditation, and breathing exercises, all of which can trigger and improve your body's relaxation response.

See also **NUTRITIONAL DEFICIENCIES, SINUSITIS, and CHAPTER 5.**

HEAD LICE

Head lice are a type of parasite skin infection that most commonly affects children, particularly young, school-age children.

Symptoms

Lice can often escape detection until the symptoms they cause become more pronounced. The most common symptom of lice infestation is persistent itching that causes children and others affected by lice to persistently scratch their heads.

Causes

Head lice can spread when other children come in contact with children already affected by lice. Lice appear as tiny, grey crawling organisms that move about on the hair and scalp. As lice infect the hair and scalp, they lay eggs or lice nits, that stick to the hair shafts close to the scalp. In appearance, lice nits are white in color. It can take between one and two weeks before lice eggs hatch to produce more lice.

Effective treatment of head lice requires a thorough approach that includes not only killing the lice and nits with special shampoo (in some cases, the heads will need to be completely shaved due to the severity of the lice infestation) and removing lice nits with a fine-tooth comb, but also thoroughly washing all clothing, towels, bed linens, and other washable materials the affected child or adult may have come in contact with, using hot water and detergent. Non-washable items, such as pillows, may require dry-cleaning, and then set aside in plastic bags for up to a week. All household and car upholstery that the affected individual may have come in contact will need to be thoroughly vacuumed, and then the vacuum bag needs to be discarded outside. Rugs and carpeting should also be thoroughly vacuumed and, ideally, steam or chem-dried. Combs, brushes, barrettes, and other hair grooming tools also need to be soaked in hot water and medicated shampoo.

In addition, since head lice is highly contagious, other people in the affected household need to be examined for lice on a daily basis for at least two to three weeks to ensure that lice does not spread. Affected individuals also need to be quarantined until their condition is fully resolved. This means avoiding all contact with the public, including going back to school during the treatment period.

Benefits

While medicated lice shampoos are the best option for killing head lice and lice nits because they act in much the same way that insecticides do, typically killing off lice and nits on contact, because of their highly toxic nature, they should only be used sparingly, no more than once a week. Between applications, daily washing of the scalp and hair (if it has not been shaved off) with an apple cider vinegar solution can enhance the benefits of lice shampoos.

ACV can help in this regard in a variety of ways.

- First, it acts as a natural *astringent* and is effective for removing dead skin cells from the scalp.

- Second, it helps to balance scalp pH so that your scalp does not become too acidic. In fact, the pH of ACV is close to the natural pH of skin, so when ACV is applied to the scalp it helps to maintain the scalp's acid mantle. This, in turn, protects against lice and lice nits, as well as foreign bacteria.

- Third, ACV helps cleanse the pores of the scalp, removing oils that may be clogging them.

- Finally, ACV helps to reduce scalp inflammation while simultaneously improve circulation in the scalp, further helping to reduce lice symptoms.

ACV Treatment

To make a topical apple cider vinegar *solution* to help treat head lice, combine one-quarter to one-third cup of ACV with one cup of warm, pure, filtered water. Mix thoroughly, then apply to your scalp and hair, massaging the mixture into all areas of your head. Let the solution sit on the scalp for at least five minutes or until it dries, then rinse your scalp and hair with water and gently towel-dry your hair. You can apply the ACV solution twice a day, morning and evening. This solution also acts as a healthy, natural hair conditioner, rinse, and shampoo.

What Else to Consider

The incidence of head lice in American children has risen in recent years. To protect your child and yourself from contracting head lice, avoid any and all areas in which head lice outbreaks may have occurred. This includes keeping your child home from school, if necessary. If you or your child does contract head lice, seek immediate medical attention and be sure to alert your local health officials, who can then inform the public and anyone you or your child may have come in contact with while infected.

See also **HAIR, DAMAGED AND DRY.**

HEARTBURN

Heartburn is the most common form of acid reflux, and is a condition that most people experience at least once in their lives. In most cases, it causes fleeting sensations of discomfort and usually resolves on its own, usually within 20 minutes to 1 to 2 hours. However, especially because of the poor eating habits of many Americans today, heartburn is becoming increasingly common, and many people experience it on a frequent, recurring basis. Severe, recurrent flare-ups of heartburn can lead to gastro-esophageal reflux disease (GERD), a serious health condition that, if left untreated, can cause esophageal (throat) cancer, a type of cancer that used to be relatively rare, but which has increased in occurrence by more than 600 percent in the U.S. over the past 30 years.

Symptoms

Symptoms commonly associated with heartburn may include:

- Burning feeling in chest
- Chest pain
- Chronic cough
- Chronic hoarseness
- Difficulty swallowing
- Sore throat

Causes

Heartburn is caused by stomach acid moving back up into the esophagus, instead of staying in the stomach where it belongs. Each time you swallow while eating or drinking, a circular muscle valve located around the bottom part of the esophagus relaxes, allowing food and liquids to pass into your stomach. Under normal conditions, once food or drink has entered your stomach, this valve, which is known as the lower esophageal sphincter, or LES, then closes to prevent stomach acid (primarily hydrochloric acid) from backing up into your throat. Heartburn occurs when the LES does not close properly, resulting in a burning sensation in the throat that can sometimes also be felt in the chest.

Benefits

Given that heartburn is caused by stomach acid backing up into the throat, it may seem odd that apple cider vinegar, which is also acidic by nature, can help relieve it. Yet, as many people have reported, very often, it can.

As I explained in the section of acid reflux, there are two possible reasons that may explain how and why ACV provides such relief. One theory is that the acetic acid in apple cider vinegar lowers stomach acidity since acetic acid is a weaker acid than hydrochloric acid. This makes sense, given that acetic acid along with its acetate salt can help buffer and maintain stomach acid at a pH level of about 3.0. At this pH range the stomach still has enough acid to digest food but not enough to trigger heartburn.

Conversely, another possible explanation lies in the theory that the LES is pH sensitive, and that when the stomach lacks enough acid to properly digest food, the LES valve does not receive the signals from the acid that cause it to close properly after swallowing. This also makes sense, since it is typically older age groups that more commonly experience heartburn. As we age, the amount of hydrochloric acid produced by our stomachs usually declines. Apple cider vinegar can supply added acid, thus providing the LES valve with the acidity signaling it needs to function properly.

ACV Treatment

If you suffer from frequent heartburn, the only way to know whether or not ACV can help you is to try it and see for yourself. To do so, add between one teaspoon to one or two tablespoons of ACV (start with the lower dose and increase if needed) to one eight-ounce glass of pure, filtered water, and drink it 20 minutes before each meal. Try to do this before every meal. If ACV is going to work with you, doing this should help prevent heartburn flare-ups or minimize their severity within a few days to a few weeks. If you do experience heartburn after you eat, you can also try drinking ACV in water when symptoms occur.

What Else to Consider

Persistent or frequently recurring heartburn can be a sign of a more serious underlying condition, such as hiatal hernia, food allergies and sensitivities, poor digestion, impaired liver function, and stomach and other gastrointestinal infections. Being overweight or obese can also cause heartburn, as can smoking, and eating overly large meals, as well as excessive protein intake, spicy foods, and foods rich in unhealthy fats.

See also **ACID REFLUX.**

HEMORRHOIDS

Hemorrhoids are characterized by inflamed, distended veins located in the lining of the anus. They can affect both children and adults and their occurrence has become so common that some physicians now regard them as normal.

Hemorrhoids can be either internal and located near the beginning of the anus, or external and located at the opening of the anus. External hemorrhoids can also protrude outside of the anus and are known as prolapsed hemorrhoids.

Symptoms

The most common symptoms of hemorrhoids are pain and discomfort following elimination and sometimes simply from sitting, anal itches, and bleeding after wiping (the blood is usually bright red).

Causes

Hemorrhoids are most commonly caused by:

- Chronic constipation
- Chronic, low-grade dehydration
- Gastrointestinal problems
- Lack of fiber-rich foods in the diet
- Nutritional deficiencies
- Poor dietary habits
- Sedentary lifestyle
- Straining during elimination

The best ways to prevent hemorrhoids and relieve their symptoms are to avoid straining during elimination, follow a diet of whole, fresh foods that includes plenty of fiber-rich foods, such as fruits, vegetables, grains and legumes; drink plenty of pure, filtered water throughout each day, and get regular exercise. These approaches can also help relieve constipation that may cause hemorrhoids or worsen their symptoms.

Benefits

Apple cider vinegar can also help relieve hemorrhoid symptoms, both when consumed and when applied topically. The pectin ACV contains can help keep your regular and make bowel eliminations easier. Moreover, many of the nutritional deficiencies that can cause hemorrhoids, such as a lack of vitamin C, B vitamins, and potassium, are also found in ACV. Because of its ability to reduce inflammation, as well as the fact that ACV acts as a natural *astringent*, topical applications of apple cider vinegar can help relieve the discomfort and pain that hemorrhoids can cause.

ACV Treatment

If you suffer from hemorrhoids, drinking one or more glasses of ACV *tonic* (one to two tablespoons of ACV combined with eight ounces of pure, filtered water) each day may help.

To make a *topical* ACV solution to treat hemorrhoids, combine equal parts of ACV and warm water. Mix together, then dip a clean cotton bowl in the solution and use to clean your anus, allowing the ACV mixture to sit on the affected area until it dries. Repeat as necessary until your pain and discomfort subsides.

What Else to Consider

Although bleeding can be a normal sign of hemorrhoids, any time that bleeding occurs you should notify you doctor or should be seen by a proctologist to rule out the existence of polyps and cancer. In some cases, hemorrhoids, especially if they are prolapsed or cause persistent pain, may require surgery. If you have prolapsed hemorrhoid or suffer from chronic hemorrhoid pain, again, consult your doctor.

See also **CONSTIPATION, GASTROINTESTINAL PROBLEMS, INFLAMMATION, and NUTRITIONAL DEFICIENCIES.**

HICCUPS

Hiccups, also spelled *hiccoughs,* are a very common, harmless yet annoying occurrence. Hiccups occur when your body's diaphragm, the muscle that separates the thoracic cavity, the part of your chest that houses your heart and lungs, from your abdomen. Your diaphragm plays an important role as you breathe, contracting each time you inhale so that air can be drawn into your lungs.

Symptoms

Hiccups are characterized as spasms of the diaphragm. As the diaphragm spasms occur and cause hiccups, they produce involuntary sounds emitted by the vocal chords. In most cases, these brief and irritable spasms resolve themselves quickly, usually no more than a few minutes. Infrequently, they can last longer.

Causes

The spasms of the diaphragm that can cause hiccups can be triggered by overeating, eating or drinking too quickly, or eating or drinking while slouching or lying down. Low stomach acid, which can lead to indigestion, can also contribute to hiccups. Most cases of hiccups can be quickly relieved simply by sitting or standing straight and drinking a glass of water. Doing so can ease diaphragm spasms. Breathing deeply into the belly can also sometimes be helpful.

Benefits

Apple cider vinegar can also help stop a bout of hiccups due to the acetic acid and other acid compounds it contains. These acids can improve the amount of stomach acid and ease diaphragm spasms.

ACV Treatment

The next time you experience a hiccup bout, try adding one to two tablespoons of ACV to eight ounces of warm, pure, filtered water. Mix thoroughly, then sip the mixture slowly. In most cases, you should experience an end to your hiccup bout within a few minutes.

What Else to Consider

To prevent hiccups, don't overeat and chew your food slowly and thoroughly. Also don't drink or eat too quickly and always avoid eating or drinking in a slouched position or while lying down. Although prolonged or frequently recurring hiccup attacks are rare, should they occur you should see your doctor.

See also INDIGESTION.

IMMUNE FUNCTION ISSUES

In order to stay healthy your body needs a strong, fully functioning immune system. It consists of a complex, interrelated network of specialized immune cells, tissues, organs, and various substances, such as enzymes and stomach acid that work together to protect against disease.

Symptoms

Symptoms of impaired immune function can vary widely, ranging from colds and congestion to fatigue, headache, and gastrointestinal problems to infections, chronic inflammation, and skin conditions.

Signs of impaired immunity can occur anywhere on or within the body. When such signs or symptoms appear, regardless of their nature, they should be immediately treated with the help of a physician.

Causes

Unfortunately, our modern lifestyle with its attendant stresses, toxic environment, and nutritionally deficient foods can often cause our immune systems to become impaired. The onset of modern devices, such as cell phones, computer laptops and tablets, smart meters, and WiFi, can further deplete immune function because of the electromagnetic frequencies (EMFs) and radiation they emit.

People who are most susceptible to impaired immune function are those with unhealthy dietary habits, nutritional deficiencies, and/or hormone imbalances, as well as those who suffer from chronic stress, fail to get enough exercise, or suffer from exposures to environmental chemicals and other toxins. As mentioned, constant exposure to WiFi, smart meters, and regular use of cell phones and other devices can also be a factor.

Benefits

Although apple cider vinegar alone is not recommended as a primary treatment for impaired immune function, ACV can help assist other treatment methods in boosting immunity and restoring your health. First, as you learned in Chapter 2, a number of scientific studies have demonstrated the ability of ACV to help fight certain infections that can suppress immune function. This is particularly true of the acetic acid in ACV, which has been shown to have potent antimicrobial properties, especially against harmful bacteria, such as E. coli bacteria (*Escherichia coli*), as well as various strains of *Salmonella*, and to inhibit the growth of bacteria on fresh fruits and vegetables. One of the reasons acetic is effective against bacteria is due to its ability to move into the cellular membranes of bacteria, causing them to die off.

Acetic acid has also been shown to also have antiviral properties. In addition, topical application of acetic acid has been shown to be effective for determining the existence of viral infections on the skin. Acetic acid's antimicrobial properties also explain why the use of ACV and other vinegars has proven so effective for helping to heal wounds. The acid compounds in ACV can also help balance and restore proper levels of stomach acid (hydrochloric acid or HCl). Adequate stomach acid levels are essential for helping to protect the gastrointestinal tract from infections.

Apple cider vinegar also aids in detoxification. Detoxification of toxins in and on the body is a very important strategy for improving immune function. ACV aids the body in detoxifying in a variety of ways, including aiding your body's bladder, gastrointestinal organs, lungs, liver, kidneys, and gallbladder functions. In addition, ACV aids in relieving constipation, helping to prevent the buildup of toxins in the GI tract. ACV also provides a variety of nutrients, fiber, enzymes, and pectin, all of which can assist your body to detoxify, while the acetic acid and other acid compounds it contains also have detoxification properties.

Finally, ACV can also help improve energy levels, making it a helpful aid for dealing with the fatigue that can often accompany impaired immune function. ACV's energizing properties are due to a number of factors. First, it contains potassium and other electrolytes, both of which are necessary for proper energy production. (Electrolytes regulate the electric charge on your body's cells and the flow of water across their membranes and also carry electrical impulses from the nerves that control your body's tissue function and movement.) The B vitamins that ACV contain are also necessary for proper energy production by your body. Moreover, ACV acts as a natural antioxidant and can help protect against free-radical damage that can cause energy loss and premature aging of your body's cell, tissues, and organs.

ACV Treatment

You can use apple cider vinegar to boost immune function in two ways, *internally and topically* for immune conditions of the skin. For *internal* infections, drink at least one glass of ACV *tonic* (one to two tablespoons of ACV added to eight ounces of pure, filtered water) each day until improvement occurs. For further benefit, you can add one tablespoon of raw, organic honey to make a *switchel tonic* (see Chapter 4, page 41), since honey also has proven immune boosting, energizing properties.

For infections anywhere on your skin, you can apply apple cider vinegar *topically* over the affected areas. Unless you have sensitive skin, there is no need to dilute the ACV. Let the ACV dry and repeat a few times each day.

What Else to Consider

To help boost your body's immune function, be sure to eat a healthy diet and avoid mucus-producing foods, such as dairy products, sugars, simple carbohydrates, and, of course, all junk foods. Instead, emphasize a diet that includes a plentiful supply of fresh fruits and vegetables (ideally organic if you can afford them), wild caught fish, free-range poultry, and whole grains.

Also be sure to stay properly hydrated each day to help your body flush out toxins and infectious bacteria, viruses, and other microbes, get regular exercise, manage your stress levels, and get enough sleep each night. For more on how to do so, see the recommendations I shared with you in Chapter 5.

While subpar immune function is increasingly common today, persistent immune issues should not be ignored, as they are often a sign of conditions that can range from chronic infections, nutrient deficiencies, and hormone imbalances, to liver disease and cancer. If you suffer from immune problems, including persistent fatigue, seek immediate medical attention.

See also **BLADDER PROBLEMS, COMMON COLDS, CONSTIPATION, CONGESTION, FATIGUE, GALLBLADDER PROBLEMS, GASTROINTESTINAL PROBLEMS, HEADACHE, INFECTIONS, INFLAMMATION, KIDNEY PROBLEMS, LIVER FUNCTION, and SKIN CONDITIONS and TOXIC OVERLOAD.**

INDIGESTION

We all experience indigestion from time to time. In most cases, indigestion is not serious, only causing fleeting sensations of discomfort that usually resolves on their own, usually within 20 minutes to a few hours.

Symptoms

Signs of indigestion may include:

- Full feeling (bloating)
- Growling stomach
- Nausea
- Upper abdomen discomfort
- Vomiting

Causes

Indigestion is usually due to one or more of the following factors:

- Drinking unhealthy beverages
- Eating unhealthy foods
- Eating when stressed or experiencing other heightened emotions (sorrow or anger)
- Enzyme and nutritional deficiencies
- Food allergies
- Overeating

In some cases, indigestion can also be caused by bacterial overgrowth in the stomach or the rest of the gastrointestinal tract, or be due to candidiasis (fungal yeast overgrowth). Indigestion may also be a symptom of acid reflux and a lack of necessary stomach acid, which is necessary to properly digest food (especially protein foods) and prevent stomach infections.

To avoid indigestion it is important to follow a diet of healthy, nutritious, fiber-rich foods, keep your body adequately hydrated, engage in regular exercise, and avoid eating meals when you are stressed or emotionally upset. Sugar, simple carbohydrates, fried foods, spicy foods, caffeine, and alcohol can also cause or contribute to indigestion, and therefore should also be avoided.

Benefits

Just as it does for acid reflux, candidiasis, and other gastrointestinal problems, apple cider vinegar can often help relieve indigestion. ACV is able to do this for a variety of reasons.

- First, ACV acts as a natural prebiotic, helping stimulate the growth of healthy bacteria in the GI tract that aid digestion and help to keep us regular, and also keep unhealthy flora such as *Candida albicans,* the yeast fungus that causes candidiasis, in check.

- Second, the compounds in ACV also act as natural enzymes, further aiding digestion.

- Third, ACV's antibacterial and antiviral properties help to prevent and reduce bacterial and viral infections in the stomach and the rest of the GI tract.

- Finally, a glass of ACV tonic before meals can help improve the level of stomach acids. Proper stomach acid levels are essential both for healthy digestion, and also for preventing infections in the stomach and the rest of the GI tract.

ACV Treatment

If you suffer from indigestion, try drinking one to three glasses of apple cider vinegar *tonic* each day (one tablespoon of ACV combined with eight ounces of pure, filtered water), ideally 20 minutes before each meal.

What Else to Consider

Chronic indigestion problems, no matter how minor they may seem, should not be ignored. If you suffer from such problems on an ongoing basis, seek prompt medical attention. Smoking, and eating overly large meals, as well as excessive protein intake, spicy foods, and foods rich in unhealthy fats can also cause indigestion. They should all be avoided.

See also **ACID REFLUX, ALLERGIES, CANDIDIASIS, and GASTROINTESTINAL PROBLEMS.**

INFECTIONS

Infections can take hold anywhere on or within the body. As they do so, the infectious microbes start to multiply and can potentially cause cellular damage as they release their toxins into the body. All types of infection, regardless of their nature, should be treated with the help of a physician.

Symptoms

Symptoms of infection can vary widely, ranging from colds and congestion to fatigue, headache, gastrointestinal problems, and sore throat. Inflammation is also typically present in cases of infection, as the inflammatory response is one of the ways in which the body deals with infection.

Causes

Infections are caused by harmful bacteria, viruses, and fungi and can be either acute or chronic in nature. People who are most susceptible to infections are those with unhealthy dietary habits, who have nutritional deficiencies, have a weakened immune system, or who suffer from chronic stress.

Benefits

Although apple cider vinegar alone is not recommended as a primary treatment for infection, ACV can help assist other treatment methods in restoring your health. As you learned in Chapter 2, a number of scientific studies have demonstrated the ability of ACV to help fight infections. This is particularly true of the acetic acid in ACV, which has been shown to have potent antimicrobial properties, especially against harmful bacteria such as E. coli bacteria (*Escherichia coli*), as well as various strains of *Salmonella*. Acetic acid vinegar has also been found to be effective for inhibiting the growth of bacteria on fresh fruits and vegetables. One of the reasons acetic is effective against bacteria is due to its ability to move into the cellular membranes of bacteria, causing them to die off.

Acetic acid has also been shown to also have antiviral properties. In addition, topical application of acetic acid has been shown to be effective for determining the existence of viral infections on the skin, which is why, as you also learned in Chapter 2, midwives in indigenous cultures in both Africa and South America use vinegar washes to screen and protect expectant mothers from the human papilloma virus (HPV). Acetic acid's antimicrobial properties also explain why the use of ACV and other vinegars has proven so effective for helping to heal wounds.

The use of ACV and other vinegars to treat infection dates back at least to the time of Hippocrates nearly 2,500 years ago. In modern times, in addition to research showing how the acetic acid in ACV and other vinegars is effective against E. coli, salmonella, and other food-borne pathogens, other studies have shown it can also help treat infections related to foot and toe nail fungus, lice, earache and ear infections, and warts.

ACV Treatment

You can use apple cider vinegar to treat infections in two ways. For internal infections, drink at least one glass of ACV *tonic* (one to two tablespoons of ACV added to eight ounces of pure, filtered water) each day until your infection clears. For further benefit, you can add one tablespoon of raw, organic honey to make a *switchel tonic* (*see* page 41), since honey also has proven infection-fighting properties.

For infections anywhere on your skin, you can apply apple cider vinegar *topically* over the affected areas. Unless you have sensitive skin, there is no need to dilute the ACV. Let the ACV dry and repeat a few times each day.

What Else to Consider

At the first sign of infection symptoms, you should see a doctor. In addition, to more quickly recover from infections avoid mucus-producing foods, such as dairy products, sugars, simple carbohydrates, and, of course, all junk foods. Instead, emphasize a diet that includes a plentiful supply of fresh fruits and vegetables (ideally organic if you can afford them), wild caught fish, free-range poultry, and whole grains, while also drinking plenty of pure, filtered water each day. Also be sure to get plenty of rest and adequate sleep and do your best to manage any stress you may be experiencing. *See* Chapter 5.

See also COMMON COLDS, CONGESTION, EAR INFECTIONS, FATIGUE, FOOT AND TOE NAIL FUNGUS, GASTROINTESTINAL PROBLEMS, HEADACHE, INFLAMMATION, LICE, SORE THROAT and WARTS.

INFLAMMATION

Inflammation is one of the ways your body responds to and goes about healing infections, as well as sprains, injuries and other types of physical trauma.

Symptoms

Signs of inflammation may be marked by:

- Fatigue
- Fever/chills
- Flu-like symptoms
- Headaches

- Joint pain, stiffness
- Redness, area may be warm to the touch
- Swollen joints

Causes

Inflammation can also be caused or made worse by a poor, nutritionally deficient diet, especially diets high in acidifying foods, such as the standard American diet.

Inflammation can occur anywhere in or on the body depending on what triggers it. Because this is so, proper treatment for inflammation can also vary. In cases of external inflammation, treatment remedies can include alternating heat and cold therapies such as heat pads and cold packs, compression bandages, splints, and keeping the affected body part elevated. Internal inflammation can often be effectively treated by following a healthy diet, the use of nutritional and appropriate herbal remedies, and, if necessary, antibiotics and anti-inflammatory drugs.

Benefits

For both external and internal inflammation, apple cider vinegar can aid in such treatments. Doing so will deliver the same anti-inflammatory nutrients and enzymes that ACV contains to the affected area.

ACV Treatment

For cases of external inflammation, you can apply an ACV *compress* to the affected area, holding it in place for 20 to 30 minutes. Doing so can help inflammation to subside as the ACV soaks into the skin, delivering the anti-inflammatory nutrients and enzymes it contains to the injured site. There is no need to dilute ACV for this purpose unless you have very sensitive skin.

For internal cases of inflammation, drink one or more glasses of ACV *tonic* (one to tablespoons of ACV added to eight ounces of pure, filtered water) each day until your conditions subside.

What Else to Consider

At the first sign of serious inflammation symptoms, as well as serious cases of physical injury, seek immediate medical attention. In addition, to more quickly recover from inflammation avoid mucus-producing foods, such as dairy products, sugars, simple carbohydrates, and, of course, all junk foods. Instead, emphasize a diet that includes a plentiful supply of fresh fruits and vegetables (ideally organic if you can afford them), wild caught fish, free-range poultry, and whole grains, while also drinking plenty of pure, filtered water each day. Also be sure to get plenty of rest and adequate sleep and do your best to manage any stress you may be experiencing.

See also **CHAPTER 5.**

INSECT BITES AND STINGS

Insect bites and stings can range in severity, from being little more than an irritating nuisance to requiring immediate medical attention in cases of anaphylactic shock and other serious allergic reactions to bites and stings.

Symptoms

Symptoms of insect bites and stings include swelling, redness, hives, itching, and pain. In some cases dizziness can also occur, as can shortness of breath. Trouble breathing after insect bites or stings can be a warning sign of anaphylactic shock and requires immediate medical attention.

Causes

Virtually any type of insect can cause bites or stings, but the ones that most commonly do so are ants, bees, hornets, spiders, and wasps.

Benefits

Applied topically, apple cider vinegar can help prevent and soothe insect bites and stings. ACV can prevent insect bites and stings due to the acetic compounds it contains. These compounds act as a natural insect deterrent, helping to keep insects away from the body. Because ACV also acts as natural *astringent* and can help reverse inflammation, it can also help relieve the swelling, redness, itching, and pain associated with insect bites and stings.

ACV Treatment

To prevent insect bites and stings you can make an apple cider vinegar *spray*. Simply add equal parts of ACV and water to a clean spray bottle and mix them together by shaking the bottle. Then spray the mixture on your face (keep it away from your eyes), arms, and other exposed skin before going outdoors.

In cases of bites and stings, you can apply undiluted apple cider vinegar directly to the affected site by soaking it in a clean cloth or towel. Hold over the affected areas for a minute or two, and repeat every 15 to 30 minutes until your symptoms ease. Not only will using ACV for this purpose help reduce inflammation, pain, redness, and itching, it can also aid your body in expelling any insect venom in your skin.

What Else to Consider

To avoid getting bit or stung by insects, avoid areas in your home and yard where insects frequent. If you have to be near such areas, cover your head and wear long sleeve shirts and pants. In cases of indoor insect infestation, you may need to seek the help of a pest control specialist. Also keep your house clean and be sure to promptly discard any leftover foodstuffs that can attract insects indoors. Making sure your windows are screened can also prevent insects from entering your home.

At the first sign of an allergic reaction following an insect bite or sting, seek immediate medical attention. If you know you are allergic to insect bites and stings, carry an epinephrine pen or an antihistamine medication with you. Also beware of insect bites and stings that don't heal normally over time, even if they seem minor. Slow healing can be a sign of nutritional deficiencies or an underlying health condition. See your doctor if bites or stings do not heal normally.

See also **INFLAMMATION and NUTRITIONAL DEFICIENCIES.**

INSOMNIA

Aside from lack of sleep itself, which has become a national epidemic, insomnia is the most common sleeping problem in the U.S. today. Approximately 60 percent of all American adults experience some degree of insomnia on a weekly basis.

Symptoms

Insomnia is characterized by an inability to either fall asleep easily or to remain asleep during the night. People with insomnia may also experience fatigue or low energy, difficulty concentrating, and mood disturbance.

Causes

Insomnia can be caused by a number of factors, ranging from psychological reasons, such as anxiety and emotional stress, to a variety of physiological issues, including poor diet, eating too close to bedtime, nutritional deficiencies, food allergies, gastrointestinal problems, chronic back or joint pain, and hormone imbalances.

Noisy nighttime environments can also cause insomnia, as can sleeping next to cell phones, plugged in electrical appliances, in homes with WiFi, or sleeping on an uncomfortable mattress. Ironically, the use of sleeping pills can also cause insomnia, as can the regular use of other pharmaceutical drugs.

Benefits

Proper treatment of insomnia requires first determining the specific factors that are keeping you from easily falling and staying asleep and then properly addressing them. For insomnia and other sleep problems, apple cider vinegar may be able to help, as well, should nutritional imbalances be a factor. That's because apple cider vinegar not only contains many of the vitamins and minerals that are necessary for obtaining deep, restful sleep, such as B vitamins and potassium, but also aids your body in better assimilating the nutrients you obtain from the foods and beverages you consume.

ACV Treatment

To see if apple cider vinegar can help improve your sleep, try drinking glass of ACV *tonic* in the evening, a few hours before bedtime. Add one to two tablespoons of ACV to eight ounces of pure, filtered water. (Avoid drinking any type of beverage just before you go to bed, as doing so may cause you to wake up during the night needing to go to the bathroom.)

What Else to Consider

To better ensure a good night's rest, follow the healthy sleep guidelines I shared in Chapter 5. While occasional insomnia is normal for most people, persistent insomnia is not. If you regularly have trouble falling and staying asleep, consult your doctor or consider working with a sleep specialist.

See also **ALLERGIES, CHRONIC BACK or JOINT PAIN, GASTROINTESTINAL PROBLEMS, HORMONE IMBALANCES, NUTRITIONAL DEFICIENCIES and SNORING.**

IRRITABLE BOWEL SYNDROME (IBS)

Irritable bowel syndrome, or IBS, is a gastrointestinal disease that affects the large intestine (colon). In most cases, IBS is a chronic condition. However, because it is not associated with inflammation of the colon or damage to the intestinal lining and tissues, unlike conditions such as ulcerative colitis and Crohn's disease, it is not a risk factor for colon and other types of cancer.

Symptoms

It is characterized by:

- Abdominal pain
- Alternating bouts of constipation
- Diarrhea
- Fatigue
- Flatulence
- Nausea

In addition, many people who suffer from IBS can manage their symptoms simply by following a healthy diet, managing stress, and making appropriate lifestyle changes.

Causes

The exact cause of IBS remains unknown. However, a number of factors are associated with IBS. Poor diet is a primary contributing factor, especially diets that lack enough fiber, include excessive and unhealthy fats, or feature sugars and refined carbohydrates. Alcohol can also trigger IBS. Other contributing factors include stress, hormone imbalances, and bacterial and viral overgrowth in the gastrointestinal tract. Nutritional deficiencies can also play a role, especially a lack of vitamin A and zinc, as can food allergies.

Benefits

While certainly not a cure, apple cider vinegar can help prevent and relieve IBS symptoms. ACV is able to do this for a variety of reasons, including because of its pectin content (pectin acts as a natural fiber). The acetic acid and other acid compounds ACV contains can also help resolve in the following ways:

- First, they act as natural prebiotics, helping stimulate the growth of healthy bacteria in the GI tract that aid digestion and help to keep us regular.
- Second, these compounds in ACV also act as natural enzymes, further aiding digestion.
- Third, ACV's antibacterial and antiviral properties help to prevent and reduce bacterial and viral infections in the stomach and the rest of the GI tract. ACV can also help prevent constipation and diarrhea that are associated with IBS.

ACV Treatment

If you suffer from IBS, try drinking one to three glasses of apple cider vinegar *tonic* each day (one tablespoon of ACV combined with eight ounces of pure, filtered water), ideally 20 minutes before each meal.

What Else to Consider

To help prevent and ease IBS symptoms it is important to follow a diet of healthy, nutritious, fiber-rich foods, keep your body adequately hydrated, engage in regular exercise, and avoid eating meals when you are stressed or emotionally upset. Sugar, simple carbohydrates, fried foods, and alcohol should also be avoided.

Persistent IBS symptoms should not be ignored. If you suffer from such problems on an ongoing basis, seek prompt medical attention.

See also **CONSTIPATION, DIARRHEA, FATIGUE, FLATULENCE, and NUTRITIONAL DEFICIENCIES.**

JOINT PAIN

Joint pain rivals back pain as being one of the most common types of both acute and chronic pain conditions. Nutritional deficiencies, including potassium, which is found in ACV, can also cause or contribute to back pain because of how these deficiencies can trigger muscle tightness and lactic acid buildup, along with impairing circulation within muscle tissues.

Symptoms

There are many body parts and many causes involved in joint pain, however there are some common symptoms, such as:

- Locking of the joint
- Redness
- Stiffness
- Swelling

- Tenderness
- Warmth
- Weakness

Causes

Joint pain can be due to sprains, injuries, and tears of joint muscles, tendons, and ligaments. It can also be due to arthritis, especially rheumatoid arthritis, an autoimmune disease that most commonly affects ligaments and tendons and joints composed of connective tissue, causing them to become inflamed and, in some cases, deformed. A sedentary lifestyle can also be a factor.

Benefits

While apple cider vinegar is not a cure for joint pain, is can help relieve joint pain symptoms. The primary way it does this is by neutralizing the buildup of acids in the body due to its alkalizing effect once it is consumed and metabolized. This, in turn, can help alleviate symptoms of inflammation in the joints.

ACV Treatment

You can use apple cider both orally and topically to help soothe joint pain. Taken as a *tonic* (one to two tablespoons of ACV added to eight ounces of pure, filtered water), it can help to reduce inflammation.

A hot apple cider *bath soak* (four to six cups of ACV added to hot bath water) can further soothe and relax joint muscles that are tight or sore. You can soak in such baths for 30 minutes or more.

What Else to Consider

To treat joint pain effectively, you need to work with a trained pain specialist, preferably one who does not regard your condition as incurable, as so many conventional doctors do. Ideally, you will want to work with a specialist not only in pain management but also with a background in dietary intervention, nutritional medicine, and detoxification. Acupuncture treatments can also be helpful, as can learning how to effectively exercise, including performing stretching exercises. (If you are unused to regular exercise, start slowly and consider initially working with a professional trainer.)

See also **ARTHRITIS and BACK PAIN.**

KIDNEY PROBLEMS

Kidney problems range from kidney infections, debris in the kidneys, kidney stones, and, in severe cases, kidney failure, a life-threatening condition that requires immediate medical. Depending on their size, kidney stones may also require medical attention, as large kidney stones (stones greater than 5 mm in size) can block the flow of urine from the kidneys through the ureters and into the bladder, causing kidney damage and other serious health problems. Kidney stone pain, regardless of kidney stone size, can also require pain medications until the stones pass or are removed by surgery or lithotripsy, a procedure which uses shock waves to shatter kidney stones so that they can more easily pass on their own.

Symptoms

Kidney problems are commonly marked by:

- Fatigue
- Feeling weak
- Pale skin
- Swelling of feet and ankles

- Loss of appetite
- Nausea

- Weight loss

Causes

Infections of the kidney are most commonly bacterial in nature, with strain of E. coli most often being the culprit. The infections can originate in the kidneys themselves or be due to bladder or other urinary tract infections that migrate into the kidneys.

Kidney stones can be caused by various factors, including poor diet, chronic, low-grade dehydration, nutritional deficiencies, especially a lack of magnesium and potassium, excess consumption of meats and other animal protein foods, and the consumption of oxalate foods, such as spinach and cabbage. (Oxalates are compounds that can interfere with the body's ability to properly assimilate calcium. The most common types of kidney stones are calcium oxalate stones.) Coffee and other caffeine drinks can also cause kidney stones. In some cases, kidney stones may be genetic in nature or be due to excessive production of parathyroid hormone by the parathyroid gland, a condition known as hyperparathyroidsim that displaces calcium into the kidneys. Lack of exercise and being overweight can also increase the risk of kidney stones.

Benefits

The primary way to prevent both kidney infections and kidney stones is to drink plenty of pure, filtered water each and every day. Doing so flushes out both infections and debris from the kidneys. Adequate water consumption, along with a healthy diet, proper nutritional supplementation, and regular exercise can significantly reduce the risk of both kidney infections and stones, and help to prevent their recurrence.

Just as it does for bladder problems and urinary tract infections, apple cider vinegar can also help, due to ACV's antiseptic and antibacterial properties, and because of the nutrients it provides, particularly magnesium and potassium, necessary minerals for healthy kidneys that can also help prevent kidney stones because of their ability to regulate calcium and keeping it from being deposited in the kidneys.

ACV Treatment

If you suffer from kidney problems, try drinking glasses of apple cider vinegar *tonic* throughout the day. Simply mix one or two tablespoons of ACV with eight ounces of pure filtered water and drink this mixture four or more times each day.

Soaking in a hot bath can also help soothe symptoms of kidney pain caused by infections or stones. An ACV *bath* can also help relax the bladder and ureter muscles, making it easier for small kidney stones, if they are present, to pass safely out of the body through urination. To make an ACV *bath* add four cups of ACV to bath water and soak for 20 to 30 minutes.

What Else to Consider

Persistent kidney problems can lead to more serious health problems. Therefore, if your problem persists, seek immediate medical attention. You may need to be prescribed a course of antibiotics in order to fully resolve your kidney problems if they are due to infection. To best ensure the health of your kidneys, also consult with a urologist on an annual basis to monitor your kidney function.

To help prevent a recurrence of kidney problems, be sure to eat a healthy diet and drink plenty of pure, filtered water throughout each day. (For more information on why diet and adequate water intake are so important, see my recommendations in Chapter 5.) You should also avoid coffee and other caffeinated drinks, alcohol, and soft drinks, and minimize your intake of meats and other animal protein foods, as well as oxalate foods, and eliminate all junk foods, sugars, refined carbohydrates, unhealthy fats, and fried foods from your diet. Getting regular exercise and, if necessary, losing weight can also be helpful.

See also BLADDER PROBLEMS, NUTRITIONAL DEFICIENCIES, OVERWEIGHT, and URINARY TRACT INFECTIONS.

LARYNGITIS

Laryngitis is a condition caused by inflammation of the larynx, or voice box, and, in some cases, inflammation of the upper windpipe (trachea).

Symptoms

The primary symptoms of laryngitis are hoarseness or loss of voice, throat rawness, a tickle in the throat, and, in some cases, a constant urge to clear the throat. Difficulty swallowing can also occur. Laryngitis is most often not serious, typically lasting for only a day or more, although it can last longer.

Causes

Laryngitis can occur on its own or be an accompanying symptom of other conditions, such as colds or flu, or be caused by bacterial or viral infections, allergies, a sore throat, or exposure to toxic chemicals in the environment. Prolonged periods of time spent in indoor environments with excessively dry air, such as during winter, can also cause laryngitis, as can overusing your voice (especially yelling or screaming) and being dehydrated. Cigarette smoking can also cause laryngitis.

Benefits

The acids and nutrients contained in ACV all have antibacterial and antiviral properties that kill infections associated with laryngitis. In addition, apple cider vinegar has an alkalizing effect within the body, meaning it helps neutralize acid buildup. This is important, since bacteria and viruses that can cause laryngitis thrive within an overly acidic environment within the body. ACV can also help thin mucus and relieve congestion associated with laryngitis. Drinking a glass of ACV tonic can also help rehydrate your body.

ACV Treatment

The best way to treat laryngitis is to avoid speaking so that your throat can heal. Drinking water with apple cider vinegar (one to two tablespoons of ACV added to eight ounces of pure, filtered water) can also help, especially when consumed at the first sign of laryngitis symptoms.

Besides drinking ACV *tonics* to help relieve laryngitis, you can also make an ACV *gargle solution.* This can be prepared in the same way as you would make an ACV *tonic.* Instead of drinking the *tonic,* use it the same way you would use a mouthwash, tilting back your head and gargling with it for a few minutes, making sure that the gargle reaches to the back of your throat. Once you are done, spit the solution out and rinse your mouth with pure, filtered water. For added benefit, you add a tablespoon of raw, organic honey to the both the ACV and *tonic solutions.* Honey will help to further soothe throat rawness and contains its own potent mix of immune-boosting nutrients.

To ease congestion associated with laryngitis, you can also use ACV as a *steam treatment* and in your bath. To make a *steam treatment,* add one cup of ACV to a pan, along with four to six cups of water. Bring the water to a boil. Once this happens, turn off the stove and cover your head with a towel, deeply inhaling the steam from the mixture. Don't force your breath and continue to breathe with your head covered until your symptoms lessen.

To prepare an ACV *bath soak,* fill your tub with water as hot as you can tolerate, and add three to four cups of ACV. Soak for 20 to 30 minutes, with your body submerged up to your neck if it is comfortable for you to do so. Inhale deeply as you soak to obtain similar benefits as those of the ACV steam.

What Else to Consider

To prevent and speed up recovery from laryngitis avoid mucus-producing foods, such as dairy products, sugars, simple carbohydrates, and, of course, all junk foods. Instead, emphasize a diet that includes a plentiful supply of fresh fruits and vegetables (ideally organic if you can afford them), wild caught fish, free-range poultry, and whole grains, while also drinking plenty of pure, filtered water each day. If your laryngitis symptoms do not improve within one week, if could be a sign of a more serious condition. For persistent and recurring laryngitis seek prompt medical attention.

See also **ALLERGIES, COLDS, INFLAMMATION, and SORE THROAT.**

LEG CRAMPS

Leg cramps can occur at any time, but they often occur at night during sleep. In some cases, leg cramps can be quite painful. Leg cramps are caused by cramping, or tightening of leg muscles, especially the calves.

Symptoms

Leg cramps often resulting in:

- Muscle cramping or aches
- Soreness
- Stiffness

Causes

A primary cause of leg cramps is the buildup of lactic acid in muscle tissues, especially after strenuous exercise or other types of physical exertion . Lactic acid is normally produced in the body by muscles as they process essential proteins and amino acids to repair themselves. During exercise and other types of physical exertion the buildup of lactic acid increases.

Nutritional deficiencies, especially a lack of potassium and electrolytes, can also cause leg cramps, along with impairing proper circulation to and within the tissues of leg muscles.

Benefits

The potassium and electrolytes found in apple cider vinegar, along with the other nutrients and acid compounds ACV contains, can help to minimize lactic acid buildup and also improve its release when muscle ache and stiffness arise.

ACV Treatment

Taken as a *tonic* (one to two tablespoons of ACV added to eight ounces of pure, filtered water), it can help to reduce inflammation associated with leg cramps. A hot apple cider *bath soak* (four to six cups of ACV added to hot bath water) can further soothe and relax leg muscles that ache, are stiff, or cramping. You can soak in such baths for 30 minutes or more.

During episodes of leg cramps, you can also apply an apple cider vinegar *compress* over the cramping area. To make an ACV *compress* combine equal parts of ACV and warm water and mix thoroughly, then soak a clean wash cloth or towel in the mixture. Apply the *compress* over the cramping area and hold in place until your symptoms subside. As the *compress* is in place, with your free hand you can also massage your leg muscles to improve circulation.

What Else to Consider

Since leg cramps can often occur following physical exercise, try to ease into your exercise program, especially if you were formerly living a sedentary lifestyle. Learning how to effectively exercise, including performing stretching exercises, is also important. (If you are unused to regular exercise, start slowly and consider initially working with a professional trainer.) Also avoid excessive physical exertion. Keeping yourself adequately hydrated is also important (*see* Proper Hydration: Your Body's Many Needs for Water in Chapter 5, page 47).

Most cases of leg cramps resolve quickly. Prolonged or recurrent cases of leg cramps, however, can sometimes be a symptom of an underlying health condition, such as fibromyalgia. If you suffer from chronic leg cramps or pains, consult with your doctor.

LIVER FUNCTION

Your liver is one of the most important organs in your body. It's also one of the most overworked. This is not surprising, when you consider all of the roles your liver plays each day to ensure your body's health. Located on the right sight of your abdomen just below your ribcage, your liver is responsible for performing over 500 essential functions. These include manufacturing bile (an entire quart each day) to break down fat, filtering out toxins and other harmful substances from the nearly 100 gallons of blood that passes through it each day, fighting infections, breaking down food, and aiding in the assimilation of vital nutrients to all of your body's trillions of cells, manufacturing important hormones, including estrogen, and testosterone, manufacturing healthy cholesterol, regulating blood levels of amino acids, glucose, and fats, and converting glucose into glycogen, an energy source for the body. Your liver also produces over 13,000 essential chemicals, while regulating more than 50,000 vital enzymes your body uses to maintain itself. In addition, it stores essential nutrients, including vitamins A, B12, D, and K, and produces urea, which plays an important role helping your body excrete nitrogen.

On top of all that, your liver is also one of your body's most important organs for detoxification of both internal waste products and external environmental pollutants. If your liver's ability to detoxify ceased, you would be dead within a matter of hours.

Symptoms

Symptoms associated with impaired liver function may be:

- Appetite loss
- Bruising easily
- Diarrhea
- Fatigue
- Jaundice
- Low platelet levels
- Nausea
- Stomach pain
- Swelling in abdomen or legs

Causes

Due to the continued proliferation of environmental toxins, along with common lifestyle factors such as poor diet, alcohol consumption, and the regular use of pharmaceutical drugs, your liver is constantly under siege. Over time, the impact of these and other factors can result in impaired liver function, setting the stage for poor health.

Benefits

Fortunately, your liver is one of the most resilient organs in your body. By supplying it with the nutrients it needs, eating a healthy diet, and periodically taking measures to detoxify your body, you can help your liver quickly rejuvenate itself so that it can most efficiently do its number one job—keeping you healthy.

Your liver acts in tandem with your gallbladder, and just as apple cider vinegar can help keep your gallbladder healthy, so too can ACV help maintain and improve proper liver function. ACV does this by supplying your liver with important nutrients and acid compounds, all of which can aid in helping it function properly and eliminate toxins.

ACV Treatment

To aid healthy liver function, drink one or two glasses of apple cider vinegar *tonic* (one to two tablespoons of ACV added to eight ounces of pure, filtered water) each day, ideally before 20 minutes before eating.

What Else to Consider

To determine the health of your liver it's best to have it assessed by your doctor, who can do so through a blood test, which should be a part of an over-all annual health checkup. If necessary, he or she can also help you create and follow a comprehensive liver rejuvenation program under his or her supervision.

To further help your liver, reduce your intake of red meat, substituting instead with wild-caught fish and lean cuts of poultry and organ meats. Additionally, stay away from poultry raised on "factory farms," choosing organically raised, free-range chicken whenever possible. And if you do choose to eat red meat, select products that come from grass-fed animals, as they are free of the antibiotics and growth hormones that are common in factory-farm meats and poultry and which place an additional burden on your liver. Overall, though, you should avoid a high-protein diet.

Also limit yourself to no more than one to two glasses of wine or beer per week. Alcohol intake places another burden on your liver, and should therefore be minimized while you are boosting your liver's health. Also be sure to refrain from drinking any other forms of alcoholic beverages, and eliminate all "junk" foods from your diet, as well as simple (white) carbohydrate foods, foods high in sugar, and any product that contains corn syrup, fructose or sucrose, as well as hydrogenated oils, all of which are unhealthy.

Finally, be sure to drink plenty of pure, filtered water each and every day, since adequate water intake is vital for proper liver function.

See also GALLBLADDER PROBLEMS, and TOXIC OVERLOAD.

METABOLISM ISSUES

Just as the incidence of fatigue has become increasingly common today, so too has a sluggish metabolism. Without a healthy metabolism, you body cannot produce all of the energy it needs, and its ability to burn fat can become impaired, leading to excessive weight gain. Impaired metabolism can also lead to the onset of serious illness. This can occur when some organs, such as your pancreas or liver no longer function correctly. In addition, cancer is increasingly being shown to be a metabolic disease. Therefore, keeping your metabolism efficient and healthy is vitally important for your overall health and vitality.

Symptoms

Signs of a sluggish metabolism may include:

- Depression
- Difficulty losing weight
- Fatigue
- Feeling cold
- Malaise—general weakness
- Pale urine
- Quick to gain weight

Causes

Conditions that may alter the metabolic rate creating a slow metabolism include:

- Age
- Diabetes
- Fasting or consuming too few calories
- Fatty tissue
- Hypothyroidism
- Low estrogen levels
- Low testosterone levels
- Medications
- Too much cortisol—Cushing's syndrome

Benefits

There are a number of things you can do to boost your metabolism. These include eating a healthy diet and avoiding consuming too many carbohydrate foods, regularly exercising, especially engaging in a combination of aerobic and strength-training exercises, keeping your body properly hydrated by drinking plenty of pure, filtered water throughout each day, avoiding unhealthy lifestyle choices, such as cigarette smoking and alcohol overconsumption, and, if necessary, losing excess weight. Getting adequate amounts of healthy, restful sleep is also very important for maintaining proper metabolic function.

ACV contains potassium and other electrolytes, both of which are necessary for proper energy production and efficient metabolic function. (Electrolytes regulate the electric charge on your body's cells and the flow of water across their membranes and also carry electrical impulses from the nerves that control your body's tissue function and movement.) The B vitamins that ACV contains are also necessary for proper energy production and metabolic function. Moreover, ACV acts as a natural antioxidant and can help protect against free-radical damage causing energy loss and impaired metabolism.

ACV Treatment

Adding a glass or more of apple cider vinegar *tonic* (one to two tablespoons of ACV combined with eight ounces of pure, filtered water) can also help boost your metabolism. ACV helps to boost metabolism in the same ways that it can help banish fatigue—by helping to improve your body's energy levels.

What Else to Consider

To improve your body's metabolic rate, be sure to eat a healthy diet, stay properly hydrated, get regular exercise, get enough sleep each night, avoid unhealthy lifestyle practices, and lose any unnecessary weight. For more on how to do so, see the recommendations I shared with you in Chapter 5.

If you suspect your metabolism is sluggish, see your doctor. An impaired metabolism can be a sign of, or contribute to, more serious underlying conditions, which can range from chronic infections, fatigue, nutrient deficiencies, and hormone imbalances, to type 2 diabetes, liver disease, obesity, and cancer.

See also CANCER, FATIGUE, HORMONE IMBALANCES, INFECTIONS, NUTRIENT DEFICIENCIES, LIVER DISEASE, OBESITY, and TYPE 2 DIABETES.

MORNING SICKNESS

Morning sickness is a fairly common condition that can affect women during pregnancy, especially during the first trimester, although in some cases it can persist throughout pregnancy. Since the symptoms of morning sickness can occur as early as two weeks after pregnancy occurs, in some cases it is the first indication a woman may have that she is pregnant.

Symptoms

The primary symptoms of morning sickness are nausea and vomiting. The name *morning sickness* is actually inaccurate because its symptoms can occur at any time of the day or night.

Causes

Morning sickness can be caused or made worse by a poor diet, nutritional deficiencies, and imbalances in the body's acid-alkaline (pH) ratio. Hormone fluctuations and imbalances, and impaired liver function and/thyroid function can also be involved.

Benefits

To prevent morning sickness during pregnancy, women are advised to eat a diet of healthy foods, with an emphasis on a plentiful supply of fresh fruits and vegetables (ideally organic if you can afford them), wild caught fish, free-range poultry, and whole grains, while also drinking plenty of pure, filtered water each day. Certain spices, especially ginger, can also help prevent and minimize morning sickness symptoms, as can, in some cases, salt on food. Greasy, fatty foods should always be avoided, as should all junk foods, sugars, and refined carbohydrates, even though some women may crave such unhealthy foods at times during pregnancy. Healthy snacks, as well as nibbling on Saltines or soda crackers can also sometimes be helpful, as can regular, moderate exercise, getting adequate sleep, and breathing fresh air.

ACV can help provide nutrients needed for health, including healthy pregnancies, and also improve the body's ability to assimilate and make use of the nutrients one receives from food and beverages. In addition, ACV helps to balance pH levels in the body, while calming the stomach, further minimizing the risk of nausea.

ACV Treatment

Sipping an apple cider vinegar *tonic* (one to two tablespoons of ACV added to eight ounces of pure, filtered water) can also help. For added benefit, you can also add a tablespoon of raw, organic honey to ACV *tonic*.

What Else to Consider

Most cases of morning sickness do not require medical attention, only rest, a healthy diet, and avoidance of anything that may trigger symptoms of nausea or vomiting. However, immediate medical attention should be sought by all pregnant women if their nausea or vomiting symptoms become severe, or if they experience difficulties keeping down liquids, feel dizzy or faint, or experience heart palpitations (racing heartbeat).

See also LIVER FUNCTION, and NUTRITIONAL DEFICIENCIES.

MUCUS BUILDUP

Mucus is produced by, and which covers, your body's mucous membranes. A certain amount of mucus is necessary for your body to function optimally because mucus contains a number of health-enhancing substances, such as antiseptic enzymes, lactoferrin (an immune compound with strong anti-microbial properties), and various other immune system antibodies, including immunoglobulins. Mucus is also necessary for protecting the epithelial cells that line the cavities and surfaces of your body's respiratory, gastro-intestinal, and urinary-genital tracts, as well as your body's visual and auditory systems.

Another primary role of mucus is to protect against infectious bacteria, viruses, and fungi. It also helps to keep your lungs healthy by trapping foreign substances that may enter them through your nose as you breathe.

Symptoms

Under normal, healthy conditions, mucus is thin and clear. When disease strikes, however, mucus can thicken and change color, appearing yellow or green as a result of its trapping bacteria or in response to viruses.

Causes

While increased mucus production is one of the ways in which your body fights infection, and when your immune system is healthy, this increased mucus production will typically run its course within a few days before returning back to normal. Prolonged, excess mucus production, however, can exacerbate the symptoms of infectious diseases, such as colds and flu, causing congestion, coughing, and possibly triggering respiratory conditions, such as asthma or bronchitis.

Benefits

Apple cider vinegar can help relieve excess mucus buildup because of its natural antihistamine effects, as well as its acid-alkaline balancing properties, and also its ability to thin mucus. You can use ACV in three ways to help minimize mucus symptoms: as a *tonic*, as part of a *steam* treatment, and as a *bath soak*.

ACV Treatment

To use as a *tonic*, combine one to two tablespoons of ACV with eight ounces of pure, filtered water. Drink one to three glasses per day.

To make a *steam* treatment, add one cup of ACV to a pan, along with four to six cups of water. Bring the water to a boil. Once this happens, turn off the stove and cover your head with a towel, deeply inhaling the steam from the mixture. Don't force your breath and continue to breathe with your head covered until your symptoms lessen.

To prepare an ACV *bath soak,* fill your tub with water, as hot as you can tolerate, and add three to four cups of ACV. Soak for 20 to 30 minutes, with your body submerged up to your neck if it is comfortable for you to do so. Inhale deeply as you soak to obtain similar benefits as those of the ACV steam. *See* also inset on Nasal Wash, page 102.

What Else to Consider

Because excess mucus production can be caused by a variety of factors, it is important to work with your doctor, who can help you to best determine the causes affecting you. I also recommend that you avoid mucus-producing foods, such as dairy products, sugars, simple carbohydrates, and, of course, all junk foods. Instead, emphasize a diet that includes a plentiful supply of fresh fruits and vegetables (ideally organic if you can afford them), wild caught fish, free-range poultry, and whole grains, while also drinking plenty of pure, filtered water each day.

MUSCLE ACHE AND STIFFNESS

Muscle ache and stiffness are extremely common, especially as people age, and among people who lead inactive, sedentary lives.

Symptoms

The muscle aches and stiffness can develop nearly anywhere in the body, such as neck, back, legs, and hands.

Causes

The primary cause of both muscle ache and muscle stiffness is the buildup of lactic acid in muscle tissues. Lactic acid is normally produced in the body as a result of muscles as they process essential proteins and amino acids to repair themselves. During exercise and other types of physical exertion the buildup of lactic acid increases, often resulting in sore, stiff muscles. This buildup can be minimized by stretching before or after such exercises or exertion. Massaging sore muscles can also help.

As with back pain, nutritional deficiencies, especially a lack of potassium and electrolytes, can also cause muscles to ache and stiffen, along with impairing proper circulation to and within muscles tissues. Muscle pain and stiffness may also be due to tension and stress.

Benefits

The potassium and electrolytes found in apple cider vinegar, along with the other nutrients and acid compounds ACV contains, can help to minimize lactic acid buildup and also improve its release when muscle ache and stiffness arise.

ACV Treatment

Taken as a *tonic* (one to two tablespoons of ACV added to eight ounces of pure, filtered water), it can help to reduce inflammation associated with muscle ache and stiff muscles.

A hot apple cider *bath soak* (four to six cups of ACV added to hot bath water) can further soothe and relax muscles that ache or are stiff or spasming. You can soak in such baths for 30 minutes or more.

What Else to Consider

Since muscle ache and stiffness most commonly occur following physical exercise, try to ease into your exercise program, especially if you were formerly living a sedentary lifestyle. Learning how to effectively exercise, including performing stretching exercises, is also important. (If you are unused to regular exercise, start slowly and consider initially working with a professional trainer.) Also avoid excessive physical exertion. Keeping yourself adequately hydrated is also important (*see* Proper Hydration: Your Body's Many Needs For Water in Chapter 5, page 47).

Most cases of muscle ache and stiffness should resolve within a few days. Prolonged muscle ache and stiffness, however, can sometimes be a symptom of an underlying health condition, such as fibromyalgia. If you suffer from chronic muscle aches or pains, consult with your doctor.

See also **BACK PAIN.**

NOSEBLEED

Nosebleed, which most commonly occurs during childhood, refers to the loss of blood from the mucous membranes that line the nose. Typically, nosebleed occurs in only one nostril.

Causes

Nosebleed can be caused by a blow to the nose, blowing one's nose too hard, scratches from fingernails, breathing excessively dry air, irritating crust formations in the nasal cavities, and nasal infections. In some cases, nutritional deficiencies may also be involved, especially a lack of vitamin C and vitamin K.

Benefits

Most cases of nosebleed are minor and usually quickly resolve. To help hasten recovery from nosebleed, first lean forward and gently blow all blood from your nose, tilt head back and breathe in and out through your mouth, pinching your lower nostrils. If bleeding does not subside within a few minutes, you can pack the affected nostril with cotton or gauze while still keeping your head tilted back and breathing through your mouth.

ACV Treatment

Soaking cotton or gauze in a solution of apple cider vinegar diluted in water (one teaspoon or more each of ACV and pure, filtered water) can be even more helpful; ACV contains both vitamins C and K, both of which help blood congeal.

What Else to Consider

Nosebleeds that do not stop after 20 minutes require medical attention, as do recurring cases of nosebleeds. Nosebleed can also be caused by aspirin or blood-thinning medications. If you experience nosebleed while using such drugs, notify your doctor. To help prevent nosebleeds, keep adequately hydrated, avoid blowing your nose too strongly, and keep your nasal cavities clear.

See also NUTRITIONAL DEFICIENCIES.

NUTRIENT ABSORPTION AND NUTRITIONAL DEFICIENCIES

In discussions about health it is often said, "You are what you eat," meaning that that foods you eat determine how healthy you are. While this is true, a more accurate statement might be, "You are what you absorb." For it's not so much the foods that we eat that make us healthy or sick, it's more whether the nutrients and other necessary compounds foods contain are able to be properly absorbed and utilized by our bodies that most matters.

Symptoms

If your body is unable to efficiently assimilate and make use of the nutrients contained in your food, the end result is nutritional deficiencies that negatively impact the literally hundreds of vital functions your body constantly performs. Symptoms indicating nutritional deficiency may include:

- Amnesia
- Anorexia
- Bruising
- Confusion

- Dementia and other neurological signs
- Growth retardation

- Loss of appetite
- Memory loss
- Weakness

Causes

Unfortunately, most people today are not able to fully absorb and make use of the vitamins, minerals, healthy fats, and other nutrients from their foods, even when they do their best to eat only healthy foods, due to a variety of factors that can impair digestion, ranging from enzyme deficiencies, gastro-intestinal problems, and others to stress or other emotional upsets while eating. All such factors can significantly diminish how well your body digests the foods you eat and is able to put the nutrients they contain to full and proper use.

Compounding the problem of impaired digestion is the fact that most people today, even those who are health conscious, fail to eat a wide variety of foods, instead routinely consuming the same, limited variety of meals over and over again. Doing so limits the array of nutrients they take in from the foods they eat.

In addition, due to many decades of large-scale, commercial farming methods, the mineral content of crop soil in which much of the food in the United States is grown has been depleted. Without an adequate amount of minerals in soil, the crops produced in the soil contain lower levels of their own nutrients than they used to. Research shows that on average American cropland has been depleted of 85 percent of its mineral content, compared with crop soil from a century earlier. Given that nutritional deficiencies and impaired nutrient absorption are both major causative factors for nearly all disease conditions, you can understand why improving your nutritional intake is so vital to your health.

Benefits

While apple cider vinegar alone is not enough to achieve healthy, stable nutritional levels, it can go a long way in helping you to do so, in large part because of the acid compounds ACV contains. These acids have the ability to improve your body's ability to more fully absorb and make use of nutrients from the foods you consume each day. In this respect, ACV's organic acids act in much the same way that enzymes do, helping your body to more easily break down food, and better assimilate and metabolize nutrients. In addition, as you learned in Chapter 2, ACV also contains a variety of nutrients important for health.

ACV Treatment

By including ACV as part of your daily diet, both as a *tonic* in water (one to two tablespoons of ACV added to eight ounces of pure, filtered water) once or twice a day, and as a *dressing* on salads and on raw and steamed vegetables, as well as eating a diet that contains a plentiful supply of mineral-rich foods, you will help your body better absorb and make use of the nutrients it needs for performing its literally hundreds of functions.

What Else to Consider

Being aware of your body's overall nutritional status is important for determining how healthy you actually are. For this reason, I recommend that you ask your doctor to assess your nutritional status as part of an annual, comprehensive health checkup. Such evaluations can easily be done via blood and urine testing.

In addition, to better ensure you are getting all of the nutrients you need to stay healthy, eat a wide variety of healthy foods, varying your meal plans beyond what you may now be used to, and making sure to eat a plentiful supply and variety of fresh fruits and vegetables, along with seeds, nuts, wholesome grains and legumes, lean meats and poultry, and wild-caught fish.

Also, chew your food thoroughly so that your body can better absorb it, and try to avoid eating when you are stressed or upset.

See also GASTROINTESTINAL PROBLEMS.

OBESITY

No pun intended, yet obesity is one of our nation's largest health problems, and trends indicate it is only growing bigger. Currently, nearly 20 percent of all children between the ages of 2 and 19 are obese, according to the latest statistics supplied by the Centers for Disease Control and Prevention (CDC), triple the rate of childhood obesity in 1980. And in adults the problem is even worse. According to the CDC 33.8 percent of all men and women in the U.S. are obese. And this trend shows no signs of reversing itself. Especially when an additional nearly 30 percent more people in the U.S. are unhealthily overweight, though not yet obese.

The obesity epidemic our nation is facing is not only tragic, it also has the potential to bankrupt the United States' healthcare system. It's long been known that obesity is directly linked to the leading causes of death in the U.S., including heart disease, stroke, hypertension, type 2 diabetes, and various types of cancer. The risk for all of these conditions rises significantly due to obesity. Obe-

sity is also a major cause of sleep apnea, osteoarthritis, depression, kidney problems, and various common gastrointestinal and respiratory conditions, along
with erectile dysfunction in men. Additionally, obesity has now surpassed
smoking to become our nation's number one cause of preventable deaths.

Causes

In order to successfully reverse this trend, we as a nation must accept a harsh
truth: *With rare exceptions, obesity is primarily the consequence of people's lifestyle
choices and eating habits.* True, there are many external factors that also play a
role in rising obesity rates, including the way that manufacturers of high-calo-
rie, high-fat, high-sugar and low-nutrient foods and beverages incessantly
target children and adolescents through the media, the proliferation of fast
food restaurants and inexpensive and unhealthy meals, the widespread use
of high-fructose corn syrup, and decades of faulty dietary advice from our
own government which, until recently, erroneously emphasized a low-fat diet
that championed carbohydrate foods. (We now know that excess carbohydrate intake, including complex carbohydrates, contribute far more to weight
gain than fats do. In fact, healthy fat intake is essential for proper metabolism
and aids in weight loss.)

But the bottom line still comes down to individual choice. No one is forc-
ing us to eat badly or to continue our increasingly sedentary lifestyles. Continuing to do so is simply inexcusable, especially in light of all of the research
proving that obesity is both preventable and reversible through healthy
choices we can all make on our own, namely eating more wisely and exercising more (*see* Chapter 5).

Benefits

While apple cider vinegar by itself is certainly no solution for weight loss, it
can serve as a weight loss aid. Its role in doing so is due to a number of factors.
One of the most important is the fact that ACV has a positive effect on the
human body's insulin response and helps to lower blood glucose (sugar) levels after meals. This fact has been demonstrated by numerous studies on apple
cider vinegar, as well as other vinegars. This same research has found that
these benefits are primarily due to ACV's acetic acid content. ACV's ability
to help manage and improve the body's insulin response is significant because
nearly all people who are overweight or obese also suffer from insulin resistance, meaning the insulin their bodies produce in response to eating is no
longer sufficient to effectively manage blood glucose levels.

Compounding this problem is the fact that, since the body cannot excrete
excess insulin, it stores the insulin as fat. This is one of the reasons why people

with insulin resistance gain weight and have a difficult time shedding it. In addition, insulin itself is a fat-storing hormone, so when it is produced in excess amount it triggers the body's other fat-storing mechanisms. People with insulin resistance can gain weight even when they eat normal amounts of calories, if the calories are from foods that trigger too much insulin production (primarily from low-fat, high-carbohydrate meals). Excess insulin can also cause you to feel hungrier, further complicating weight loss.

Additional research has shown that the acetic acid in ACV and other vinegars can reduce the glycemic index (GI) of foods by as much as 30 to 35 percent. The glycemic index indicates the effects of a particular food on blood sugar levels. The higher the glycemic index of a food is, the more that food will cause a spike in blood sugar levels after it is consumed. High glycemic foods also contribute to unhealthy weight gain, including by triggering the hunger response even after one has eaten shortly before.

According to Carol S. Johnston, Ph.D, R.D., Professor and Associate Director of the Nutrition Program in the School of Nutrition and Health Promotion at Arizona State University, the acetic acid in ACV and other vinegars prevents a percentage of starchy, high GI foods from being digested and raising blood sugar levels, adding that its effects are similar in nature to blood sugar medications. Research has also shown that consuming vinegar before bedtime can also reduce blood glucose levels during the night.

Finally, research has also shown that drinking a glass of water containing apple cider vinegar before or after meals can increase feelings of satiety (fullness). When we feel full, we are likely to consume less food during each day, and therefore less calories.

Although there are very few studies that have researched the potential benefits of vinegar for weight loss, one such study did show some benefit. The study was conducted by researchers in Japan and involved 175 participants, all of whom were obese but otherwise healthy. Over the course of 12 weeks, the participants consumed either vinegar (between half an ounce to one ounce per day) or water each day and consumed similar diets. They also kept a food journal. At the end of the study, the vinegar group had lost slightly more weight than the control group. While the weight loss itself was not significant (on average only one to two additional pounds compared to that of the control group), what was noteworthy was that the vinegar group also showed improvements (reductions) in their triglycerides levels. (Elevated triglycerides increase the risk of heart disease and stroke.) Moreover, the overall body fat mass of the vinegar group also showed notable improvement. While the vinegar used in this study was not ACV, its benefits were primarily due to the acetic acid in the vinegar which, of course, ACV also contains.

ACV Treatment

Given the above benefits that ACV and other vinegar are known to have for improving some of the mechanisms associated with unhealthy weight gain, it makes sense to drink one to three glasses of ACV *tonic* per day (one table-spoon of ACV added to eight ounces of pure, filtered water) if you are trying to lose weight or if you want to avoid gaining excess pounds.

What Else to Consider

It bears repeating: Apple cider vinegar alone is far from enough to achieve significant weight loss. An effective weight loss program involves a combination of following a healthy diet that limits your intake of carbohydrates and other high glycemic foods, adequate hydration, and regular exercise. Other factors, such as hormone imbalances, food allergies, and chronic stress, which can lead to emotional eating, can also need to be addressed.

If you are overweight or obese, take action now to lose weight by working with your doctor. Also avoid the quick-fix promises of fad diets and so-called "magic bullet" supplements and drugs. Simply put, they don't work, are a waste of money, and may make you weight condition even worse.

PSORIASIS

Psoriasis is a skin condition that usually affects the outside of the knees, elbows, scalp, and lower back. Children get psoriasis, but it is most common in adults.

Symptoms

It is characterized by thick, reddish patching of the skin. The patches may sometimes also be covered with silvery scales. Unlike other skin conditions, psoriasis typically does not itch.

Causes

Psoriasis can caused by one or more of the following factors: food and/or environmental allergies, poor diet, nutritional deficiencies, low stomach acid (hydrochloric acid, or HCl), or chemical exposures. Excessive secretions of oily fatty acids onto the skin can also cause or exacerbate psoriasis due to bacterial overgrowth that such acids can trigger. Bacteria thrive on skin that is overly acidic and oily. Chronic stress and emotional upset can exacerbate psoriasis conditions.

Benefits

Apple cider vinegar applied topically to the skin, can help minimize and eliminate psoriasis problems. ACV acts as a psoriasis remedy in a number of ways.

- First, it acts as a natural astringent and is effective for removing dead skin cells from the skin.

- Second, it helps to balance skin pH so that your skin does not become too acidic. In fact, the pH of ACV is close to the natural pH of skin, so when ACV is applied to skin it helps to maintain the skin's acid mantle. This, in turn, protects against foreign bacteria.

- Third, ACV helps cleanse the pores of the skin, removing oils that may be clogging them.

- Finally, ACV helps to reduce scalp inflammation while simultaneously improve circulation in the skin.

ACV Treatment

Treatment of psoriasis should be overseen by a dermatologist. Working with a physician with a background in nutritional medicine and allergies can also be helpful. Commercial shampoos and related hair care products that contain irritating chemicals should also be avoided.

To make a *topical* psoriasis solution using apple cider vinegar, combine one-quarter to one-third cup of ACV with one cup of warm, pure, filtered water. Mix thoroughly, then soak a clean, cotton wash cloth or towel in the mixture. Apply the cloth or towel to the affected, holding it in place for 20 to 30 minutes. Repeat as necessary, or least once a day (morning and evenings).

Drinking one or more glasses of apple cider vinegar *tonic* can also sometimes help heal psoriasis because of its acetic acid content, which can help improve stomach acid levels. As we age, the amount of hydrochloric acid produced by our stomachs usually declines. Apple cider vinegar supplies added acid to the stomach, helping cases of psoriasis where HCl deficiencies are a causative factor. If you suffer from psoriasis, combine one or two tablespoons of ACV to one eight-ounce glass of pure, filtered water, and drink it 20 minutes before each meal. Try to do this before every meal.

What Else to Consider

Since psoriasis problems can be caused or made worse by an overly acidic condition due to one's diet, if you continue to experience psoriasis problems consider consulting with a nutritionally-trained physician or certified clinical nutritionist who can help your create a healthier, more akalizing diet (*also see* the dietary recommendations in Chapter 5, beginning on page 43).

To avoid bacterial overgrowth on your skin, bathe or shower regularly, wear clean clothes, and avoid the use of chemically-laden soaps and other body cleansing and hair care products.

See also ALLERGIES, SKIN CONDITION, NUTRITIONAL DEFICIENCIES, and SKIN CONDITIONS.

RASHES

Rashes are a type of skin condition that is most often minor and temporary. It is an area of irritated or swollen skin that can develop instantly or over a number of days.

Symptoms

Most rashes present as eruptions on the skin that are reddish, inflamed, and usually cause itching. The skin may become dry and scaly or fluid-filled blisters may form.

Causes

Rashes can be caused by one or more of the following factors:

- Food and/or environmental allergies
- Poor diet
- Nutritional deficiencies
- Low stomach acid (hydrochloric acid, or HCL)
- Chemical exposures

Excessive secretions of oily fatty acids onto the skin can also cause or exacerbate rashes due to bacterial overgrowth that such acids can trigger. Bacteria thrive on skin that is overly acidic and oily.

Benefits

Apple cider vinegar applied topically to the skin can help minimize and eliminate rashes. ACV acts as remedy for rashes in a number of ways.

- First, it acts as a natural *astringent* and is effective for removing dead skin cells from the skin.
- Second, it helps to balance skin pH so that your skin does not become too acidic. In fact, the pH of ACV is close to the natural pH of skin, so when

ACV is applied to skin it helps to maintain the skin's acid mantle. This, in turn, protects against foreign bacteria.

- Third, ACV helps cleanse the pores of the skin, removing oils that may be clogging them.

- Finally, ACV helps to reduce inflammation associated with rashes while simultaneously improving circulation in the skin.

ACV Treatment

Treatment of persistent rashes should be overseen by a dermatologist. Working with a physician with a background in nutritional medicine and allergies can also be helpful. Commercial shampoos and related hair care products that contain irritating chemicals should also be avoided.

To make a *topical* rash solution using apple cider vinegar, combine onequarter to one-third cup of ACV with one cup of warm, pure, filtered water. Mix thoroughly, then soak a clean, cotton wash cloth or towel in the mixture. Apply the cloth or towel to the affected, holding it in place for 20 to 30 minutes. Repeat as necessary, or least once a day (morning and evenings).

Drinking one or more glasses of apple cider vinegar *tonic* can also sometimes help heal rashes because of its acetic acid content, which can help improve stomach acid levels. As we age, the amount of hydrochloric acid produced by our stomachs usually declines. Apple cider vinegar supplies added acid to the stomach, helping cases of rashes where HCl deficiencies are a causative factor. If you suffer from rashes, combine one or two tablespoons of ACV to one eight-ounce glass of pure, filtered water, and drink it 20 minutes before each meal. Try to do this before every meal.

What Else to Consider

Since rashes can be caused or made worse by an overly acidic condition due to one's diet, if you continue to experience rashes consider consulting with a nutritionally-trained physician or certified clinical nutritionist who can help your create a healthier, more alkalizing diet (*also see* the dietary recommendations in Chapter 5, beginning on page 43).

To avoid bacterial overgrowth on your skin, bathe or shower regularly, wear clean clothes, and avoid the use of chemically-laden soaps and other body cleansing and hair care products.

See also **ALLERGIES, NUTRITIONAL DEFICIENCIES, and SKIN CONDITIONS.**

SCALP PROBLEMS

Although the most common scalp problem is dandruff, some people may also be affected by other scalp problems, such as scalp itch, scalp rashes, or an excessively oily scalp. Most often, such conditions are caused by the same factors that cause dandruff.

Symptoms

Scalp problems can be uncomfortable and is characterized by a variety of symptoms, including:

- Blisters
- Bumps
- Flakiness
- Hair loss
- Itchiness
- Rashes
- Sores

The symptoms may vary in severity.

Causes

Primarily, the cause of scalp problems includes scalp inflammation accompanied by excessive secretions of oily fatty acids onto the scalp and bacterial overgrowth on the scalp. Such bacteria can thrive on scalps that are overly acidic and oily. Other common causes of scalp problems are commercial shampoos and related hair care products that contain irritating chemicals.

Benefits

Apple cider vinegar, applied topically to the scalp, can help minimize and eliminate scalp problems. ACV acts as a scalp remedy in a number of ways.

- First, it acts as a natural *astringent* and is effective for removing dead skin cells from the scalp.
- Second, it helps to balance scalp pH so that your scalp does not become too acidic. In fact, the pH of ACV is close to the natural pH of skin, so when ACV is applied to scalp it helps to maintain the the scalp's acid mantle. This, in turn, protects against foreign bacteria.
- Third, ACV helps cleanse the pores of the scalp, removing oils that may be clogging them.
- Finally, ACV helps to reduce scalp inflammation while simultaneously improve circulation in the scalp, further helping to reduce scalp problems.

To make a *topical* scalp solution using apple cider vinegar, combine one-quarter to one-third cup of ACV with one cup of warm, pure, filtered water. Mix thoroughly, then apply to your scalp and hair, massaging the mixture into all areas of your scalp. Let the solution sit on the scalp for at least five minutes or until it dries, then rinse your scalp or hair with water and gently towel-dry your hair. You can apply the ACV solution twice a day, morning and evening. This solution also acts as a healthy, natural hair conditioner, rinse, and shampoo.

What Else to Consider

Since scalp problems are most commonly caused by an overly acidic condition due to one's diet, if you continue to experience scalp problems, consider consulting with a nutritionally-trained physician or certified clinical nutritionist who can help your create a healthier, more alkalizing diet (also see the dietary recommendations in Chapter 5, beginning on page 00). To avoid bacterial overgrowth on your scalp, wash your scalp and hair regularly, and avoid the use of chemically-laden shampoos and other hair care products.

See also **DANDRUFF, HAIR, DAMAGED AND DRY.**

SHINGLES

Shingles is a painful skin rash. Those most at risk of developing shingles after they've had chickenpox are people over 50 years of age (the risk increases even more after age 70), and people whose immune systems are weak. Most cases of shingles last between two to six weeks.

Symptoms

Shingles outbreaks can occur anywhere on the body, but primarily occur on the arms or the upper torso, appearing as a string of rash-like blisters. While not a life-threatening condition, shingles can be a persistent condition and the pain it can cause can be severe and debilitating. Pain is usually the first indication of shingles, and can cause sensations of burning, numbness, and tingling. Within a few days, the pain is followed by a red rash that can then start to blister and crust over. Aside from the pain shingles causes, other symptoms can include itching, fever, and fatigue.

In certain cases, shingles can result in other serious health problems, including vision loss if shingles occurs near the eyes, and lingering nerve pain (neuralgia) even after the shingles rash disappears due to the nerve damage shingles can cause. Depending on which nerves are affected, shingles can also cause other neurological conditions, including facial paralysis, hearing problems, troubles with balance, and even inflammation of the brain (encephalitis). Lingering skin conditions can also incur due to bacterial infections.

Causes

This painful condition is caused by the varicella-zoster virus, which is the same virus that causes chickenpox. In people who experienced chicken pox, the virus can lay dormant in nerve tissues near your spinal cord and brain, only to be reactivated years later. It is this reactivation of the virus that causes shingles. The use of the prednisone and other steroid medications can also increase the risk of shingles.

Benefits

There is no known cure for shingles. Conventional medical treatments for it can include antiviral drugs, pain medications, and local anesthetics. To prevent shingles, physicians recommend getting either the chickenpox vaccine or, for people 60 and older, the shingles vaccine. Neither vaccine is a treatment for shingles after it has occurred, however, nor are the vaccines a guarantee that a shingles outbreak will not still occur after receiving them. Both vaccines can also cause side effects.

In addition to the drug treatments above, physicians also recommend that people with shingles regularly take baths and apply cool, wet compresses over the affected part of the body with shingles in order to help relieve pain and itching. Both of these measures can be enhanced by the use of apple cider vinegar. Not only will using apple cider vinegar improve the ability of baths and compresses to soothe shingles' symptoms, ACV's proven antiviral properties can help speed recovery of shingles as ACV comes in contact with the affected area. Keep in mind, however, that ACV is most definitely not a cure for shingles.

ACV Treatment

To use ACV in your *bath*, add three to four cups of ACV to bath water and then soak in the bath for 20 to 30 minutes. To make an ACV *compress*, combine equal parts of ACV and cold or room temperature water and mix together. Then soak a clean wash cloth or towel in the mixture and apply it over the area of your body with shingles, holding it in place for 30 minutes. You can repeat the use of ACV *baths* and *compresses* more than once each day.

What Else to Consider

At the first sign of shingles, seek immediate medical attention, and most especially if shingles pain or rash occurs near your eyes (if left untreated, shingles infection can lead to permanent eye damage), if you are over age 70, or if you have a weakened immune system due to suffering from other chronic health conditions and/or are taking medications that can suppress immune function. To improve your recovery from shingles, avoid mucus-producing foods, such as dairy products, sugars, simple carbohydrates, and, of course, all junk foods. Instead, emphasize a diet that includes a plentiful supply of fresh fruits and vegetables (ideally organic if you can afford them), wild caught fish, free-range poultry, and whole grains, while also drinking plenty of pure, filtered water each day. You may also want to consider receiving acupuncture treatments, due to acupuncture's proven ability to relieve pain, including nerve pain.

See also **FATIGUE, RASH, and SKIN CONDITIONS.**

SINUSITIS

Sinusitis is a disease in which the cavities around the nasal passages become inflamed. Sinusitis can either be acute (short-term) or chronic, as well as recurring.

Symptoms

Symptoms of sinusitis include:

- Diminished sense of smell
- Facial pain
- Fatigue
- Head congestion

- Headache
- Laryngitis
- Postnasal drip
- Runny nose

Causes

Sinusitis is a condition caused by infection in the sinuses. The infections can be bacterial, viral, or fungal. When such infections take hold in the sinuses, they cause the mucous membranes that line them to become inflamed. In addition to infections, various other factors can trigger sinusitis, including tobacco smoke, extremely dry or cold air, and air pollutants and irritants in one's home or place of work. Food allergies and acid reflux can also cause or contribute to sinusitis, as can poor diet, nutritional deficiencies, and impaired immune function.

Benefits

Like colds and flu, which are also infectious disease, in the case of sinusitis it is not the infections themselves that determine whether or not sinus infections will develop. Rather, it depends on the health of your immune system and whether or not your body is in a state of chronic, low-grade acidity due to your diet. Sinus infections thrive in an overly acidic environment within the body.

It is because of these two factors that apple cider vinegar can help prevent and relieve sinusitis symptoms. First, the acids and nutrients contained in ACV all have immune-enhancing, antibacterial, antifungal, and antiviral properties. Second, when taken orally, apple cider vinegar has an alkalizing effect within the body, meaning it helps neutralize acid buildup. Just as importantly, ACV's ingredients work together to help thin mucus so that the body can rid itself of excess mucus more easily. ACV also acts as a natural anti-inflammatory agent, which can help alleviate inflammation associated with sinusitis and sinus congestion in general.

ACV Treatment

To help relieve sinusitis symptoms, drink at least one glass of apple cider vinegar *tonic* (one to two tablespoons of ACV added to eight ounces of pure, filtered water) per day. Drinking three or four glasses of ACV *tonic* per day will help even more.

To further ease sinusitis symptoms, you can also use ACV as a *steam* treatment and in your bath. To make a *steam* treatment, add one cup of ACV to a pan, along with four to six cups of water. Bring the water to a boil. Once this happens, turn off the stove and cover your head with a towel, deeply inhaling the steam from the mixture. Don't force your breath and continue to breathe with your head covered until your symptoms lessen.

To prepare an ACV *bath soak*, fill your tub with water as hot as you can tolerate, and add three to four cups of ACV. Soak for 20 to 30 minutes, with your body submerged up to your neck if it is comfortable for you to do so. Inhale deeply as you soak to obtain similar benefits as those of the ACV steam.

What Else to Consider

To improve your recovery from sinusitis, avoid mucus-producing foods, such as dairy products, sugars, simple carbohydrates, and, of course, all junk foods. Instead, emphasize a diet that includes a plentiful supply of fresh fruits and vegetables (ideally organic if you can afford them), wild caught fish, free-range poultry, and whole grains, while also drinking plenty of pure, filtered water each day. For persistent or recurring sinusitis, seek prompt medical attention.

See also **ACID REFLUX, ALLERGIES, COLDS, and LARYNGITIS.**

SKIN CONDITIONS

Skin conditions affect most people from time to time, and can range from minor blemishes to acne and age spots to eczema, psoriasis, and other types of rashes. Bruising and cuts can also affect the skin.

Symptoms

Whatever irritates, inflames, or clogs your skin can result in symptoms such as swelling, redness, itching, burning, and rashes.

Causes

Overall, most skin problems are caused by inflammation accompanied by excessive secretions of oily fatty acids of the skin, which can lead to bacterial overgrowth on the skin. Such bacteria can thrive on overly acidic and oily environments. Other common causes of skin problems include one or more of the following factors: food and/or environmental allergies, poor diet, nutritional deficiencies, low stomach acid (hydrochloric acid, or HCl), or chemical exposures. Commercial shampoos and skin care products that contain irritating chemicals can also cause skin problems.

Benefits

Minor skin problems will often resolve on their own, while serious cases of skin problems should be overseen by a dermatologist. Working with a physician with a background in nutritional medicine and allergies can also be helpful.

Apple cider vinegar applied topically to the skin can help minimize and eliminate many minor skin problems, as well as more serious conditions, such as eczema, psoriasis, minor degree burns, and sunburns. ACV acts as skin remedy in a number of ways.

- First, it acts as a natural *astringent* and is effective for removing dead skin cells from the skin.

- Second, it helps to balance skin pH so that your skin does not become too acidic. In fact, the pH of ACV is close to the natural pH of skin, so when ACV is applied to skin it helps to maintain the skin's acid mantle. This, in turn, protects against foreign bacteria.

- Third, ACV helps cleanse the pores of the skin, removing oils that may be clogging them.

- Finally, ACV helps to reduce scalp inflammation while simultaneously improving circulation in the skin.

To make a topical scalp solution using apple cider vinegar, combine one-quarter to one-third cup of ACV with one cup of warm, pure, filtered water. Mix thoroughly, then apply to your skin with a clean, cotton wash cloth or cotton swab and let the solution sit on the skin until it dries, then gently rinse your skin with water and towel-dry. You can apply the ACV solution twice a day, morning and evening.

What Else to Consider

Since skin problems can be caused or made worse by an overly acidic condition due to one's diet, if you continue to experience skin problems, no matter how minor they may seem, consider consulting with a nutritionally-trained physician or certified clinical nutritionist who can help your create a healthier, more akalizing diet (also see the dietary recommendations in Chapter 5, beginning on page 43).

To avoid bacterial overgrowth on your skin, bathe or shower regularly, wear clean clothes, and avoid the use of chemically-laden soaps and other body cleansing and hair care products.

See also **ACNE, AGE SPOTS, ALLERGIES, BRUISING, BURNS, CUTS, DIET, HAIR, DAMAGED AND DRY, ECZEMA, NUTRITIONAL DEFICIENCY, PSORIASIS, RASHES, SUNBURNS, and TOXIC OVERLOAD.**

SORE THROAT

A sore throat can occur on its own or be an accompanying symptom of other conditions, such as colds, flu, strep throat, or tonsillitis. It can also be the side effect of strained vocal cords.

Symptoms

Symptoms of a sore throat can include pain and rawness, hoarseness, difficulty swallowing, congestion, and postnasal drip. Rarely are sore throats serious, and they typically last for only a few days to a week or more.

Causes

Sore throats occur because of inflammation in the throat. They can be caused by bacterial or viral infections, allergies, or exposure to toxic chemicals in the environment. Prolonged periods of time spent in indoor environments with excessively dry air, such as during winter, can also cause a sore throat, as can overusing your voice, or being dehydrated.

Benefits

The best way to treat a sore throat is to do so at the first sign of sore throat symptoms. Apple cider vinegar is an excellent home remedy for doing so. The acids and nutrients contained in ACV all have immune-boosting. antibacterial and antiviral properties. In addition, when taken orally, apple cider vinegar has an alkalizing effect within the body, meaning it helps neutralize acid buildup. This is important, since bacteria and viruses that can cause sore throat thrive within an overly acidic environment within the body. ACV can also help thin mucus and relieve congestion associated with sore throats. Drinking a glass of ACV tonic can also help rehydrate your body.

ACV Treatment

You can use apple cider vinegar in a number of ways to help banish a sore throat. At the first sign of a sore throat I recommend that you drink at least one glass of apple cider vinegar *tonic* (one to two tablespoons of ACV added to eight ounces of pure, filtered water) per day. Drinking more than one glass of ACV *tonic* per day will help even more. Doing so will help boost your body's immune function and improve its acid-alkaline balance.

In addition, I recommend you make an ACV *gargle solution.* This can be prepared in the same way as you would make an ACV *tonic.* Instead of drinking the *tonic,* use it the same way you would use a mouthwash, tilting back your head and gargling with it for a few minutes, making sure that the gargle reaches to the back of your throat. Once you are done, spit the solution out and rinse your mouth with pure, filtered water. For added benefit, you add a tablespoon of raw, organic honey to both the ACV *gargle* and *tonic* solutions. Honey will help to further soothe a sore throat and contains its own potent mix of immune-boosting nutrients.

To ease congestion associated with a sore throat, you can also use ACV as a *steam* treatment and in your bath. To make a *steam* treatment, add one cup of ACV to a pan, along with four to six cups of water. Bring the water to a boil. Once this happens, turn off the stove and cover your head with a towel, deeply inhaling the steam from the mixture. Don't force your breath and continue to breathe with your head covered until your symptoms lessen.

To prepare an ACV *bath soak,* fill your tub with water as hot as you can tolerate, and add three to four cups of ACV. Soak for 20 to 30 minutes, with your body submerged up to your neck if it is comfortable for you to do so. Inhale deeply as you soak to obtain similar benefits as those of the ACV *steam.*

What Else to Consider

To prevent and speed up recovery from a sore throat avoid mucus-producing foods, such as dairy products, sugars, simple carbohydrates, and, of course, all junk foods. Instead, emphasize a diet that includes a plentiful supply of fresh fruits and vegetables (ideally organic if you can afford them), wild caught fish, free-range poultry, and whole grains, while also drinking plenty of pure, filtered water each day. If your sore throat symptoms do not improve within one week, if could be a sign of a more serious condition. For persistent sore throats and sore throats that recur often, seek prompt medical attention.

See also **ALLERGIES, COLD, IMMUNITY FUNCTION ISSUES, INFLAMMATION, and LARYNGITIS.**

STOMACHACHE

Mostly likely everyone has experienced a stomachache at one time. In most cases, stomachache is not serious, only causing fleeting sensations of discomfort that usually resolves on their own, usually within 20 minutes to 1 to 2 hours.

Symptoms

More intense abdominal pain may be result in:

- Dehydration
- Difficult bowel movements
- Fever
- Frequent urination
- Stomach is tender to the touch
- Vomiting

Causes

Stomachaches are usually due to one or more of the following factors: eating unhealthy foods or drinking unhealthy beverages, overeating, food allergies, and enzyme and nutritional deficiencies. Stomachache can also be caused by bacterial overgrowth in the stomach or the rest of the gastrointestinal tract, or be due to candidiasis (fungal yeast overgrowth). In some cases, it can also be a symptom of acid reflux and a lack of necessary stomach acid, which is necessary to properly digest food (especially protein foods) and prevent stomach infections. Because of the poor eating habits of many Americans today, stomachaches are becoming increasingly common and many people experience them on a frequent basis.

Benefits

To avoid stomachache it is important to follow a diet of healthy, nutritious, fiber-rich foods, keep your body adequately hydrated, engage in regular exercise, and avoid eating meals when you are stressed or emotionally upset. Sugar, simple carbohydrates, fried foods, spicy foods, caffeine, and alcohol can also cause or contribute to stomachache, and therefore should also be avoided.

Just as it does for acid reflux, candidiasis, and other gastrointestinal problems, apple cider vinegar can often help relieve stomachache. ACV is able to do this for a variety of reasons.

- First, ACV acts as a natural prebiotic, helping stimulate the growth of healthy bacteria in the GI tract that aid digestion and help to keep us regular, and also keep unhealthy flora such as *Candida albicans*, the yeast fungus that causes candidiasis, in check.

- Second, the compounds in ACV also act as natural enzymes, further aiding digestion.

- Third, ACV's antibacterial and antiviral properties help to prevent and reduce bacterial and viral infections in the stomach and the rest of the GI tract.

- Finally, a glass of ACV tonic before meals can help improve the level of stomach acids. Proper stomach acid levels are essential both for healthy digestion, but also for preventing infections in the stomach and the rest of the GI tract.

ACV Treatment

If you suffer from stomachache, try drinking one to three glasses of apple cider vinegar *tonic* each day (one tablespoon of ACV combined with eight ounces of pure, filtered water), ideally 20 minutes before each meal.

What Else to Consider

Chronic stomachache problems, no matter how minor they may seem, should not be ignored. If you suffer from such problems on an ongoing basis, seek prompt medical attention. Smoking and eating overly large meals, as well as excessive protein intake, spicy foods, and foods rich in unhealthy fats can also cause stomachache. They should all be avoided.

See also **ACID REFLUX, ALLERGIES, CANDIDIASIS, GASTROINTESTINAL PROBLEMS.**

STUFFY NOSE

A stuffy nose, or nasal congestion is usually a symptom of colds, flu, or sinusitis, a disease caused by infection in the sinuses. When such infections take hold in the sinuses, they cause the mucous membranes that line them to become inflamed.

Symptoms

Stuffy nose symptoms can include:

- Diminished sense of smell
- Facial pain
- Fatigue
- Headache
- Postnasal drip
- Runny nose laryngitis

Causes

Stuffy nose is primarily caused by infections, which can be bacterial, viral, or fungal. In addition to infections, various other factors can trigger a stuffy nose, including tobacco smoke, extremely dry or cold air, and air pollutants and irritants in one's home or place of work. Food allergies can also cause or contribute to sinusitis, as can poor diet, nutritional deficiencies, and impaired immune function.

Benefits

To effectively treat a stuffy nose, it is important to also treat the underlying conditions that may be associated with it. If those conditions are infectious in nature, it is not the infections themselves that determine whether or not sinus infections will develop. Rather, it depends on the health of your immune system and whether or not your body is in a state of chronic, low-grade acidity due to your diet. Sinus infections thrive in an overly acidic environment within the body.

It is because of these two factors that apple cider vinegar can help prevent and relieve a stuffy nose. First, the acids and nutrients contained in ACV all have immune-enhancing, antibacterial, antiviral, and antifungal properties. Second, when taken orally, apple cider vinegar has an alkalizing effect within the body, meaning it helps neutralize acid buildup. Just as importantly, ACV's ingredients work together to help thin mucus so that the body can rid itself of excess mucus more easily. ACV also acts as a natural anti-inflammatory agent, which can help alleviate inflammation associated with a stuffy nose and sinus congestion in general.

ACV Treatment

To help relieve a stuffy nose, drink at least one glass of apple cider vinegar *tonic* (one to two tablespoons of ACV added to eight ounces of pure, filtered water) per day. Drinking three or four glasses of ACV *tonic* per day will help even more.

To further ease stuffy nose symptoms, you can also use ACV as a *steam* treatment and in your bath. To make a *steam* treatment, add one cup of ACV to a pan, along with four to six cups of water. Bring the water to a boil. Once this happens, turn off the stove and cover your head with a towel, deeply inhaling the steam from the mixture. Don't force your breath and continue to breathe with your head covered until your symptoms lessen. (*See* also inset on Nasal Wash, page 102).

To prepare an ACV *bath soak*, fill your tub with water as hot as you can tolerate, and add three to four cups of ACV. Soak for 20 to 30 minutes, with your body submerged up to your neck if it is comfortable for you to do so. Inhale deeply as you soak to obtain similar benefits as those of the ACV *steam*.

What Else to Consider

To further improve your recovery from a stuffy nose, avoid mucus-producing foods, such as dairy products, sugars, simple carbohydrates, and, of course, all junk foods. Instead, emphasize a diet that includes a plentiful supply of fresh fruits and vegetables (ideally organic if you can afford them), wild caught fish, free-range poultry, and whole grains, while also drinking plenty of pure, filtered water each day. For persistent or recurring stuffy nose problems, seek prompt medical attention.

See also **ALLERGIES, COLDS, FLU, LARYNGITIS and SINUSITIS.**

SUNBURN

Sunburn is caused by prolonged sunlight exposure. The affected skin area will turn color, from mildly reddish to severely red and darker. As sunburn heals, the affected skin area typically peels.

Symptoms

Depending on the severity of sunburn, symptoms can vary from mild pain, to severe pain, blistering, and swelling. Cases of sunburn are classified as first degree sunburn (mild reddening of the skin), second degree sunburn (swelling, increased pain, and blistering), and third degree sunburn, which can cause severe damage to the skin and increase the risk of skin infection.

Third degree sunburns require prompt medical attention, as do cases of second degree sunburn that show no signs of healing after a few days. In some cases, sunburn, especially if recurring, can lead to melanoma and other types of skin cancer.

Causes

Sunburns are specifically caused by overexposure to the sun's ultraviolet (UV) radiation, causing skin to become inflamed, accompanied by a usually mild burning sensation.

Benefits

The best treatment for sunburn, of course, is to avoid prolonged exposure to sunlight, especially during peak sun hours (noon to three PM). While many physicians and other health experts still continue to advise that people use UV-protecting sunscreens, the latest research suggests that such sunscreens, not sunlight exposure itself, may actually cause skin cancer, because of how important sunlight is for the production of vitamin D in the body. Vitamin D not only helps prevent melanoma and other skin cancers, it also protects against various other types of cancer, and is essential for protecting against many other serious diseases, as well, and also vital for the proper functioning of many processes in the body.

Because of how important vitamin D is to overall health, vitamin D supplements and drugs have become increasingly popular and more frequently prescribed by doctors and other health practitioners in recent years. However, the best way to ensure adequate vitamin D levels in the body remains adequate sunlight exposure (early morning sunlight exposure for 20 to 30 minutes each day is most ideal). Moreover, vitamin D supplements can cause health problems when taken in excess, including displacing calcium into the arteries, leading to atherosclerosis (hardening of the arteries), and the kidneys, thus increasing the risk of kidney stones. It's telling too that many indigenous people around the world who regularly expose most of their bodies to sunlight throughout the day have a much lower level of cancer than do people in Western and other modern cultures where people primarily spend their lives indoors.

That said, let's look at how apple cider vinegar can help relieve sunburn symptoms. It is able to do so for many of the same reasons that it can be so effective for treating scalp and other skin conditions when applied topically.

- First, it acts as a natural *astringent* and is effective for removing dead skin cells from the skin.

- Second, it helps to balance skin pH. In fact, the pH of ACV is close to the natural pH of skin, so when ACV is applied to skin it helps to maintain the skin's acid mantle. This, in turn, helps prevent foreign bacteria attacking sunburn areas and causing infection.

- Third, ACV helps cleanse skin pores and helps to reduce skin inflammation caused by sunburn while simultaneously improving circulation to the skin.

- Finally, ACV's ingredients can help protect against free radical damage caused by sunburn, not only speeding the healing of sunburn, but also protecting against skin cancer.

ACV Treatment

To make a *topical scalp solution* using apple cider vinegar, combine one-quarter to one-third cup of ACV with one cup of warm, pure, filtered water. Mix thoroughly, then apply to the affected area and surrounding skin area, gently massaging the mixture into them. Let the solution remain on the skin until it dries. You can apply the ACV solution twice a day, morning and evening.

What Else to Consider

As mentioned, second and third degree cases of sunburn should be treated by a health professional. To prevent sunburn, avoid sunlight exposure between noon and 3 PM, and wear protective headgear. While sunburn is healing avoid the use of chemically-laden soaps and other skin-cleansing products.

See also **KIDNEY PROBLEMS and SKIN CONDITIONS.**

TEETH, DISCOLORATION

Tooth discoloration occurs when the outer layer of the tooth, the enamel, is stained or when the inner structure of the tooth darkens or yellows. Tooth discoloration can also be age-related, and tooth stains may result in embarrassment.

Causes

Various factors can cause teeth discoloration. Wine, cola, coffee, certain drinks and foods, as well as habitual smoking can stain the teeth over a period of time. The thinning of the tooth enamel and poor oral care may also make teeth appear yellow.

Benefits

Just as apple cider vinegar solutions can help improve the health of your gums and bad breath, they can also be helpful as a teeth whitener. Such solutions provide a safe and inexpensive alternative to commercial teeth whitening methods, which can not only be expensive, but in many cases also involve chemicals that can cause teeth to become sensitive and pose other possible health risks as well.

ACV Treatment

To whiten your teeth using apple cider vinegar do the following:

- First, floss your gums, to loosen any debris that may be trapped between your teeth. Then rinse your mouth thoroughly.

- Next, combine equal measures of ACV and water and mix them together thoroughly. Then take a small amount of this mixture and swish it in your mouth for 30 to 60 seconds, making sure that the mixture covers all of your upper and lower teeth as you do so. Once you are done swishing, spit the mixture out, and soak your toothbrush in the remaining mixture.

- Now brush your teeth thoroughly, just as you would using toothpaste, again making sure that you cover all of your teeth. When you finish, rinse your toothbrush off and then brush your teeth again using toothpaste.

- Finish by once more swishing your mouth with the ACV mixture for another 30 to 60 seconds. If you use this method, you will likely notice improvements in your teeth within a few days or week.

   Do **NOT** *use ACV alone for the above methods. Doing so can harm your teeth by stripping away tooth enamel.*

What Else to Consider

As with all dental issues, when it comes to the appearance of your teeth, you should see your dentist regularly, ideally every six months to once a year.

See also **BAD BREATH and GINGIVITIS.**

TOXIC OVERLOAD

Toxic substances can be found in our foods, water supply, air, and even in the clothing we wear. These toxins can take the form of chemical compounds and heavy metals. While they may enter our body in very small amounts, unless our body eliminates these substances, over time the amount of these toxins buildup and play havoc with our organs.

It is therefore understandable that ongoing detoxification by your body is one of the most important ways by which it maintains its health. Your body's detoxification system, which includes the kidneys, bladder, liver, intestines, lungs, sweat glands, and the lymphatic system, works nonstop to neutralize and eliminate toxins. By doing so, it helps minimize the risk of disease, prevents damage to your body's tissues and organs, aids digestion and elimination, and improves your body's ability to make use of vital nutrients in the foods and drinks you consume.

Symptoms

Symptoms or signs that may indicate that you are possibly surrounded by too many toxins may include:

- Brain fog
- Constipation
- Dizziness
- Muscle aches and joint pains
- Ongoing fatigue
- Skin problems—acne, rashes
- Weight gain

Causes

Today, the body's detoxification system faces a herculean task for the simple fact that we live in an ever increasing toxic world, given the plethora of toxic chemicals and pollutants in the world's air, water, and soil. As a result, the ability of the body to detoxify is, in most people, impaired to some degree. As a result, most of us, suffer from some level of toxic overload, and thus we have an increase risk of becoming ill and/or aging prematurely. It's for this reason that the literally hundreds of holistic, integrative physicians, and other health practitioners it's been my good fortune to meet, interview, and learn from over the years do all they can to improve their patients' ability to detoxify. As they do so, inevitably, their health improves.

A comprehensive detoxification plan is best undertaken with the help and under the supervision of a physician or other health practitioner with a background in detoxification therapies. Still, there is much that you can do on your own to improve the functioning of your body's detoxification organs. Such measures include eating as healthily as possible, with a focus on organic foods whenever possible, and avoiding all junk foods and commercially packaged foods. Doing so will help minimize your intake of pesticides, herbicides, and other toxic chemicals that are so commonly found in our nation's food supply. Also be sure to drink only pure, filtered water, not tap water. You should also consider using a shower filter, since the many toxins that are found in most municipal water supplies are absorbed by the skin when we shower and bathe. Also avoid commercial cosmetic and household cleaning products, most of which are also toxic to some degree.

Deep breathing exercises can also help, as they aid the lungs in discharging toxins and irritants, as can regular exercise, which better enables toxins to be eliminated through the skin as you sweat. (Most people are unaware that skin is the body's largest organ of detoxification.)

You can also experiment with fasting (ideally under your doctor's supervision.) One of the easiest ways to fast is to simply not eat for one 24 hour period each month to give your body a chance to use the energy it normally expends on digestion and metabolism to detoxify instead. Should you undertake such a fast, be sure to drink a plentiful supply of pure, filtered water throughout the day. Organic, herbal teas can also help, as can fresh-squeezed vegetable juices. The next morning, break your fast gently, starting your day with another glass of water, tea or juice, and then having fruit for breakfast. For lunch, follow with soup and salad, and eat your first full meal later that day.

Benefits

Apple cider vinegar can also help improve your body's ability to detoxify. It does so in a variety of ways, including aiding your body's bladder, gastro-intestinal organs, lungs, liver, kidneys, and gallbladder functions. In addition, ACV aids in relieving constipation, helping to prevent the buildup of toxins in the GI tract. ACV also provides a variety of nutrients, fiber, enzymes, and pectin, all of which can assist your body to detoxify, while the acetic acid and other acid compounds it contains also have detoxification properties.

ACV Treatment

To aid your body in detoxifying, drink one or two glasses of apple cider vine-gar *tonic* (one to two tablespoons of ACV added to eight ounces of pure, filtered water) each day, ideally before breakfast and again a few hours before you go to bed.

What Else to Consider

To determine the health of your body's detoxification organs it's best to have them assessed by your doctor, who can do so through blood and urine tests. Then he or she can also help you create and follow a comprehensive detoxi-fication plan under his or her supervision.

See also **BLADDER PROBLEMS, CONSTIPATION, GALLBLADDER PROBLEMS, GASTROINTESTINAL PROBLEMS, LIVER FUNCTION,** and **KIDNEY PROBLEMS.**

URINARY TRACT INFECTIONS

Urinary tract infections, known as UTIs, are more common in women than men. The urinary tract is made up of the bladder, kidneys, ureters, and uretha. A UTI is an infection of any part of this system.

Symptoms

Symptoms of UTIs include:

- Blood in the urine
- Burning sensation during urination
- Change in the frequency in which you urinate
- Pain in back
- Pain in the bladder or ureter
- Pain or pressure in lower abdomen
- Volume of urine output

Causes

Urinary tract infections are caused by the buildup of bacterial infections, such as various strains of E. coli, within the urinary tract, which runs from the kidneys into the bladder. UTIs typically occur when bacteria enter the urinary tract through the urethra and begin to multiply in the bladder. Although your body's urinary system is designed to keep out such bacteria, sometimes its defenses fail, allowing bacteria to take hold and grow into a full-blown infection in the urinary tract. UTIs can also be caused by the presence of stones or gravel in the kidneys. Kidney stones and gravel can be a breeding ground for harmful bacteria, which can then migrate further down the urinary tract.

Benefits

Apple cider vinegar can often provide some degree of relief for urinary tract infections and prevent their recurrence, due to ACV's antiseptic and antibacterial properties. As I mentioned earlier, according to noted health expert Earl Mindell, ACV can also help to prevent and possibly even reverse bladder infections because of its ability to increase the acidity within the environment of the bladder and urinary tract, along with the acidity of the urine. This, in turn, helps to prevent and reverse bacterial overgrowth.

ACV Treatment

If you suffer from urinary tract infections, try drinking glasses of apple cider vinegar *tonic* throughout the day. Simply mix one or two tablespoons of ACV with eight ounces of pure filtered water and drink this mixture four or more times each day.

Soak in a hot *bath* can also help soothe symptoms of urinary tract infections by helping to relax the bladder and ureter muscles. For added benefit, you can add four cups of ACV to your *bath* and soak for 20 to 30 minutes.

What Else to Consider

Persistent urinary tract infections lasting more than a few days can lead to more serious health problems. Therefore, if your problem persists, seek immediate medical attention. You may need to be prescribed a course of antibiotics in order to fully resolve your problem.

To help prevent urinary tract infections, be sure to eat a healthy diet and drink plenty of pure, filtered water throughout each day. (For more information on why diet and adequate water intake are so important, *see* my recommendations in Chapter 5.) You should also avoid coffee and other caffeinated drinks, alcohol, 'soft drinks, and citrus juices until your urinary tract infection has cleared, as these can cause additional irritation within your urinary tract and further aggravate your symptoms.

VARICOSE VEINS

Varicose veins affect at least 30 percent of all Americans, occurring primarily in women. They are veins that develop into enlarged and twisted veins.

Symptoms

In appearance, they are typically bluish or otherwise discolored and can be hard to the touch and bulge above the rest of the skin surface in the areas of the body in which they occur (primarily the legs, although they also occur in the feet and ankles and other areas).

Causes

They are caused by blood pooling in the veins, primarily due to a lack of circulation, a sedentary lifestyle, standing for long periods of time, and lifestyle factors, such as smoking and being overweight. Nutritional deficiencies and hormonal factors (especially hormonal fluctuations that occur during pregnancy and menopause) can also cause varicose veins.

Benefits

Treatment options for varicose range from wearing support or compression stockings to lifestyle changes, such as losing weight and stopping smoking, to more involved procedures, including laser and pulsed light therapies, radiofrequency occlusion (a procedure in which a catheter is inserted into the affected vein or veins, through which radiofrequency is then delivered to the vein walls, causing the veins to heal, collapse, or close), and various other surgical methods.

Apple cider vinegar can also help reduce varicose veins. ACV does so by helping improve blood circulation and reducing inflammation.

ACV Treatment

You can use ACV in two ways to treat varicose veins, *topically* and as a *tonic*. To use *topically,* combine equal measures of ACV and water and mix them together. Then soak a wash cloth in the mixture. Apply the wash cloth directly to the affected area and hold in place for 20 to 30 minutes. To enhance this method, you can also apply heat over the wash cloth using a heating pad. This will help the ACV to penetrate deeper into the skin.

In addition to the topical method, consume at least one glass of ACV *tonic* (one to two tablespoons of ACV added to eight ounces of pure, filtered water) each day. Continue using both methods until you see improvement.

What Else to Consider

Although varicose veins are harmless, they can be an indication of nutritional imbalances or other aspects of your overall health that need attention. To determine if such factors exist consult with your doctor. Also try to avoid prolonged periods of sitting and standing.

WARTS

Warts are quite common. Other than being a nuisance, most warts are harmless tumors of the skin.

Symptoms

Warts appear as bumps of growths anywhere on the skin (most commonly on the face, scalp, fingers, knees, or elbows), and can occur singly or in clusters. Essentially, warts are benign (noncancerous) tumors and they can occur in a variety of shapes and sizes. The most common type of wart is well-defined, round, hard to the touch, and sometimes discolored in appearance.

Causes

Warts are caused by a class of virus known as the human papilloma virus (HPV), and the people who are most susceptible to them are those who suffer from nutritional deficiencies and a weakened immune system. Poor diet and poor hygiene habits can also contribute to wart growth.

Benefits

Not all warts need to be treated as, over time, they may sometimes disappear on their own as a person's immune function improves. The most common over-the-counter wart treatment is a solution containing salicyclic acid, a compound related to common aspirin that is applied topically to break down the hardened outer layer of warts and increase skin moisture. Professional care treatments include medications such as retinoid creams, cryotherapy, a process that freezes the wart usually with liquid nitrogen, causing it to eventually fall off, electrosurgery, a process in which the wart is burnt using an electrical charge, surgical removal, and chemical peels.

Fortunately, apple cider vinegar can often offer a simple, safer alternative to such treatments. ACV can help treat warts because of the acid compounds it contains, especially acetic acid, which has proven antiviral properties that are capable of killing HPV and other viruses on contact. Moreover, ACV also acts as a natural *antiseptic*.

ACV Treatment

To use ACV to treat warts, simply apply it directly to the wart then cover it with a bandage. Leave the bandage on overnight, then clean the wart in the morning and repeat the process with a new bandage. Continue this process until you see improvement, which will usually happen within a few weeks, although in some cases it may take longer. For added benefit, you can also drink one or more glasses of ACV *tonic* each day to help boost your body's immune function.

What Else to Consider

As mentioned, warts typically occur in people who suffer from nutritional deficiencies, poor diet, and suboptimal immune function. If you suffer from warts, especially if they reoccur, consult with your doctor to determine how you can improve these factors. Also be sure to practice healthy hygiene habits.

WEIGHT DISORDER

See OBESITY.

YEAST INFECTIONS

Although localized yeast infections more commonly affect women, they can affect men, as well. Such infections are caused by yeast overgrowth on or within (tongue, urinary tract, and vagina) localized areas of the body.

Symptoms

Signs of localized yeast infections can include burning, itching, a frequent urge to urinate, and unpleasant discharges from the urinogenital tract.

Causes

Like candidiasis, localized yeast infections are caused by the overgrowth of a specific yeast called *Candida albicans*, which exists in all of us and is part of the various intestinal flora that harmlessly reside in the lower intestinal tract, on our skin, and, in women, within the vagina. In healthy individuals, Candida is kept in check by a variety of healthy bacteria that also inhabit the human body. But when the balance between healthy bacteria and other flora becomes disrupted, Candida growth increases. As it does so, Candida can transform from a harmless, simple form of yeast into a more aggressive yeast fungus capable of spreading beyond where it normally occurs in and on the body.

Also like candidiasis, yeast infections most commonly strike people who eat a diet high in sugars, simple carbohydrates, and processed foods, people who suffer from nutritional deficiencies, people with a weakened immune system, people who regularly use broad spectrum antibiotic drugs (these kill off healthy flora in the GI tract), people who excessively consume alcohol (especially beer, which contains yeast), people with hormonal imbalances, and women who use birth control pills or who have undergone synthetic estrogen replacement therapy.

Benefits

Unlike candidiasis, which can take time to develop and spread, localized yeast infections can occur rapidly, and usually requires a comprehensive treatment plan in order to fully resolve it, including, if necessary, antibiotic/antifungal drugs.

Just as it can be helpful as an aid for treating candidiasis, apple cider vinegar can often enhance the effectiveness of treatments for localized yeast infections when consumed as an ACV tonic or applied topically to yeast overgrowth. ACV's benefits for treating yeast infections derive from the acetic acid and natural enzymes it contains, all of which can help regulate the growth of Candida yeast in the body. Additionally, apple cider vinegar also helps check yeast overgrowth because of its overall alkalizing effects when it is consumed. Like all other types of harmful microbes, the Candida yeast thrives in an overly acidic environment. Regular consumption of ACV in water helps to raise the pH level of such environments. Additionally, once consumed, apple cider vinegar acts as a healthy prebiotic, stimulating the growth of healthy bacteria in your gut that can further bring unhealthy flora back in check.

ACV Treatment

To augment an overall yeast treatment plan, I recommend drinking three glasses of apple cider vinegar *tonic* each day, ideally 20 minutes or more before breakfast, lunch, and dinner. For each glass, add one tablespoon of ACV to eight ounces of pure, filtered water or you can try filling a water bottle with ACV and water and sip it throughout the day.

For yeast infections on your skin, you can apply apple cider vinegar *topically* over the affected areas. Unless you have sensitive skin, there is no need to dilute the ACV. You can also soak in an ACV *bath*. Simply add three to four cups of ACV to a comfortable, hot bath and soak for 20 to 30 minutes once a day.

What Else to Consider

To properly treat yeast infections, you need to work with a health professional who knows how to most effectively deal with it. Most cases of localized yeast infections, when properly treated, resolve fairly quickly. Persistent yeast infections, however, may be a symptom of a more serious condition, including not only candidiasis but also a weakened immune system. If your infection persists, please see your doctor.

See also **CANDIDIASIS.**

Conclusion

Congratulations! By reading this far, you now know how and why apple cider vinegar can truly be called Nature's most versatile and powerful remedy. More importantly you now know how you can use apple cider vinegar to help prevent and relieve many of today's most common health problems and health risks, as well as having the knowledge you need to create an overall daily health routine.

The next step is up to you. It is not enough to know about apple cider vinegar's many benefits and the rest of the information I've shared with you. Such knowledge is of little worth unless it is applied.

Will you do so?

I sincerely hope so.

If you do, I encourage you to experiment. There is no such thing as a "one-size fits all" prescription when it comes to health and healing, and that includes the use of apple cider vinegar. Only you can determine the degree to which ACV can improve your health, and how much ACV you need to use to get the benefits you are seeking. I, for example, enjoy adding a full two tablespoons of apple cider vinegar to a glass of pure, fil-tered water. I usually drink two glasses of ACV tonic each day, along with using ACV liberally on salads and steamed vegetables. I find that works well for me.

What works well for you may be different. The only way to know is to try using apple cider vinegar in some of the ways this book suggests and see what happens. As I promised you at the very beginning of this book, if you do so I think you will find that adding ACV to your life will prove helpful to your overall health.

ACV is not a cure-all, of course, and to truly be healthy requires a more complete dedication to making healthy choices each and every day. That is why I included all of the information I did in Chapter 5. By paying attention to your overall diet, exercising regularly and wisely, keeping your body hydrated, getting enough sleep, and managing your stress levels, along with adding apple cider vinegar as a part of your daily self-care regimen, you truly will be taking steps to greater, lasting health. I wish you speedy progress along your journey.

Health and Blessings!

Resources

The following companies manufacture and supply high quality brands of raw, organic, unfiltered, pasteurized apple cider vinegar with "the mother."

Bragg's Organic Apple Cider Vinegar
Bragg Live Foods, Inc.
Box 7
Santa Barbara, CA 93102
(800) 446-1990
www.bragg.com

Complete Natural Products
1265 West 1275 North Suite #7
Centerville, UT 84014
(888) 648-4442
http://completenaturalproducts.com

Dynamic Health Organic Raw Apple Cider Vinegar
Dynamic Health Laboratories, Inc
110 Bridge Street, Suite 2
Brooklyn, NY 11201
(800) 396-2114
www.dynamichealth.com

Eden Foods Organic Apple Cider Vinegar
Eden Foods
701 Tecumseh Road
Clinton, MI 49236
(888) 424-3336
www.edenfoods.com

Omega Nutrition Certified Organic Apple Cider Vinegar
Omega Nutrition Canada
1695 Franklin Street
Vancouver, BC, Canada V5L 1P5
(800) 661-3529
www.omeganutrition.com

Simply Nature Organic Apple Cider Vinegar
(This product is produced and marketed by the international store chain, Aldi, under Aldi's exclusive Simply Nature brand. It is available at Aldi stores across the USA.)
ALDI, Inc.
1200 N. Kirk Road
Batavia, IL 60510
www.aldi.us

Spectrum Organic Apple Cider Vinegar
Spectrum Organics
The Hain Celestial Group, Inc.
4600 Sleepytime Drive
Boulder, CO 80301
(800) 434-4246
www.spectrumorganics.com

Vermont Village Organic Apple Cider Vinegar
Vermont Village Artisan Cannery
698 South Barre Road
Barre, VT, 05641
(802) 479-2558
www.vermontvillageapplesauce.com

Vitacost Organic Apple Cider
Available online from
www.vitacost.com.
Vitacost, Inc
The Kroger Co.

1014 Vine Street
Cincinnati, OH 45202
(800) 381-0759

Vitamin Shoppe Organic Apple Cider Vinegar
Available online from
www.vitaminshoppe.com.
The Vitamin Shoppe
2101 91st Street
North Bergen, NJ 07047
(866) 293-3367

The following companies manufacture and supply high quality brands of raw, organic, unfiltered, pasteurized apple cider vinegar switchel products.

Up Mountain Switchel
Up Mountain Switchel
South Londonberry, VT
Bushwick, Brooklyn, NY
www.drinkswitchel.com
info@drinkswitchel.com

Vermont Switchel
Vermont Switchel Company
PO Box 17
Hardwick, VT 05843
(802) 522-5898
www.vtswitchel.com

References

Chapter 1

Flaws, Bob. *The Tao of Healing: Dietary Wisdom According to Chinese Medicine,* 2nd ed. Boulder, CO, Blue Poppy Press, 2013.

Li Bing-shen et al. *The Treatment of Hundreds of Diseases with Vinegar & Eggs.* Shanghai,China. Shanghai Science & Technology Publishing Co., 1992.

Solieria, Laura and Giudici, Paolo, editors. *Vinegars of the World.* New York, Springer, 2009.

Chapter 2

http://bloodjournalhematologylibrary.org/content/91/10/3527.full.html. *Flavonoid-rich apples and nitrate-rich spinach augment nitric oxide status and improve endothelial function in healthy men and women: a randomized controlled trial,* July 2012

www.ncbi.nlm.gov/pubmed/19476292. *An apple a day may hold colorectal cancer at bay: recent evidence from a case-control study,* July 2012.

https://www.yahoo.com/news/m/ba4d6af2-5e3c-3c95-bd27-16c654ca8524/apple-cider-vinegar-helps.html?.tsrc=fauxdal

Chapter 3

Dirty Dozen: EWG's 2016 Shopper's Guide to Pesticides in Produce. Environmental Working Group. https://www.ewg.org/foodnews/dirty_dozen_list.php

Part Two

www.aaaai.org/about-aaaai/newsroom/allergy-statistics

Americans Spend More on Hair Care Than Dental Care. California Dental Group, March 24, 2015. www.cadentalgroup.com/americans-spend-more-on-hair-care-than-dental-care.

The Beauty Business: Pots of Promise. *The Economist,* 2003. www.economist.com/node/1795852.

Abe K, Kushibiki T, Matsue H. 2007. "Generation of antitumor active neutral medium-sized [alpha]-glycan in apple vinegar fermentation." *Biosci Biotechnol Biochem* 71:2124–29.

Adams MR. 1985. Vinegar. In: Wood BJB, editor. *Microbiology of fermented foods*. New York: IFT Press. p 1–45.

Alonso AM, Castro R, Rodriguez MC, Guillen DA, Barroso CG. 2004. "Study of the antioxidant power of brandies and vinegars derived from Sherry wines and correlation with their content in polyphenols." *Food Res Intl* 37:715–21.

Bartowsky EJ, Henschke PA. 2008. "Acetic acid bacteria spoilage of bottled red wine; a review." *Int J Food Microbiol* 125:60–70.

Beheshti, Z. et al. "Influence of apple cider vinegar on blood lipids." *Life Science Journal* 2012;9 (4).

Bjornsdottir K, Breidit JF, McFeeters RF. 2006. "Protective effect of organic acids on survival of Escherichia coli O157:H7 in acidic environments." *Appl Environ Microbiol* 72:660–4.

Blackburn CV, McClure PJ. 2002. "Modeling the growth, survival and death of bacterial pathogens in food, Kinetic growth models." In: Blackburn CV, editor. *Foodborne pathogens*. New York: Wood Head Publishing, p 56–72.

Brighenti F, Castellani G, Benini L, Leopardi E, Crovetti R, Testolin G. 1995. "Effect of neutralized and native vinegar on blood glucose and acetate responses to a mixed meal in healthy subjects." *Eur J Clin Nutr* 49:242–7.

Brul S, Coote P. 1999. "Preservative agents in foods: mode of action and microbial resistance mechanism." *Intl J Food Microbiol* 50:1–17.

Budak HB, Guzel-Seydim ZB. 2010. "Antioxidant activity and phenolic content of wine vinegars produced by two different techniques." *J Sci Food Agric* 90:2021–6.

Budak HN. 2010. *A research on compositional and functional properties of vinegars produced from apple and grape [PhD thesis]*. 190p. Isparta, Turkey: Suleyman Demirel University.

Budak HN et al. 2011. "Effects of apple cider vinegars produced with different techniques on blood lipids in high-cholesterol-fed rats." *J Agric Food Chem* 59:6638–644.

Caligiani A, Acquotti D, Palla G, Bocchi V. 2007. "Identification and quantification of the main organic components of vinegars by high resolution H NMR spectroscopy." *Anal Chim Acta* 585:110–19.

Callejón RM, Tesfaye W, Torija MJ, Mas A, Troncoso AM, Morales ML. 2008. "HPLC determination of amino acids with AQC derivatization in vinegars along submerged and surface acetifications and its relation to the microbiota." *Eur Food Res Technol* 227:93–102.

Chan E, Ahmed TM, Wang M, Chan JCM. 1993. "History of medicine and nephrology in Asia." *Am J Nephrol* 14:295–301.

Chang J, Fang TJ. 2007. "Survival of Escherichia coli O157:H7 and Salmonella enterica serovars typhimurium in iceberg lettuce and the antimicrobial effect of rice vinegar against E. coli O157:H7." *Food Microbiol* 24:745–51.

Cheng HY, Ye RC, Chou CC. 2003. "Increased acid tolerance of Escherichia coli O157:H7 by acid adaptation time and conditions of acid challenge." *Food Res Intl* 36:49–56.

Davalos A, Bartolome B, Gomez-Cordoves C. 2005. "Antioxidant properties of commercial grape juices and vinegars." *Food Chem* 93:325–30.

Ebihara K, Nakajima A. 1988. "Effect of acetic acid and vinegar on blood glucose and insulin responses to orally administered sucrose and starch." *Agric Biol Chem* 52:311–2.

Entani E, Asai M, Tsujihata S, Tsukamoto Y, Ohta M. 1998. "Antibacterial action of vinegar against food-borne pathogenic bacteria including Escherichia coli O157:H7." *J Food Prot* 61:953–9.

Escudero ME, Velazquez L, Di Genaro MS, Guzman MS. 1999. "Effectiveness of various disinfectants in the elimination of Yersinia enterocolitica on fresh lettuce." *J Food Prot* 62:665–9.

Fushimi T, Sato Y. 2005. "Effect of acetic acid feeding on the circadian changes in glycogen and metabolites of glucose and lipid in liver and skeletal muscle of rats." *Br J Nutr* 94:714–9.

Fushimi T et al. 2002. "The efficacy of acetic acid for glycogen repletion in rat skeletal muscle after exercise." *Intl J Sports Med* 23:218–22.

Fushimi T et al. 2006. "Dietary acetic acid reduces serum cholesterol and triacylglycerols in rats fed a cholesterol-rich diet." *Br J Nutr* 95:916–24.

Gullo M, Caggia C, De Vero L, Giudici P. 2006. "Characterization of acetic acid bacteria in 'traditional balsamic vinegar'." *Int J Food Microbiol* 106:209–12.

Honsho S, Sugiyama A, Takahara A, Satoh Y, Nakamura Y, Hashimoto K. 2005. "A red wine vinegar beverage can inhibit the rennin-angiotensin system: experimental evidence in vivo." *Biol Pharm Bull* 28:1208–10.

Johnston CS, Buller AJ. 2005. "Vinegar and peanut products as complementary foods to reduce postprandial glycemia." *J Am Diet Assoc* 105:1939–42.

Johnston CS. 2006a. "Strategies for healthy weight loss: From vitamin C to the glycemic response." *J Am Coll Nutr* 25:158–65.

Johnston CS. 2006b. "Vinegar: medicinal uses and antiglycemic effect." *Med Gen Med* 8:61–78.

Johnston, CS, Gaas CA. 2006. "Vinegar: medicinal uses and antiglycemic effect." *Med Gen Med.* 8(2): 61.

Johnston CS, Kim CM, Buller AJ. 2004." Vinegar improves insulin sensitivity to a high-carbohydrate meal in subjects with insulin resistance or type 2 diabetes." *Diabetes Care;* 2004 27:281–282.

Johnston CS et al. "Vinegar ingestion at mealtime reduced fasting blood glucose concentrations in healthy adults at risk for type 2 diabetes." *J of Functional Foods;* 2013. 5(4):2007-11.

Johnston CS and White, AM. "Vinegar ingestion at bedtime moderates waking glucose concentrations in adults with well-controlled type 2 diabetes." *Diabetes Care* 2007 Nov; 30(11): 2814-2815.

Kondo S, Tayama K, Tsukamoto Y, Ikeda K, Yamori Y. 2001b. "Antihypertensive effects of acetic acid and vinegar on spontaneously hypertensive rats." *Biosci Biotechnol Biochem* 65:2690–4.

Kondo T, et al. "Vinegar intake reduces body weight, body fat mass, and serum triglyceride levels in obese Japanese subjects." *Biosci. Biotechnol Biochem.* 2009 Aug;73(8):1837-43. Epub 2009 Aug 7.

Laranjinha JA, Almeida LM, Madeira VM. 1994. "Reactivity of dietary phenolic acids with peroxyl radicals: antioxidant activity upon low density lipoprotein peroxidation." *Biochem Pharmacol* 48:487–94.

Lee M, Park YB, Moon S, Bok SH, Kim D, Ha T, Jeong T, Jeong K, Choi M. 2007. "Hypocholesterolemic and antioxidant properties of 3-(4-hydroxyl) propanoic acid derivatives in high-cholesterol fed rats." *Chem Biol Interact* 170:9–19.

Leeman M, Ostman E, Bjorck I. 2005. "Vinegar dressing and cold storage of potatoes lowers postprandial glycaemic and insulinaemic responses in healthy subjects." *Eur J Clin Nutr* 59:1266–71.

Liljeberg H, Fjorck I. 1998. "Delayed gastric emptying rate may explain improved glycaemia in healthy subjects to a starchy meal with added vinegar." *Eur J Clin Nutr* 52:368–71.

Marler JB et al. "Human health, the nutritional quality of harvested food and sustainable farming systems." *Nutritionsecurity.org.* www.nutritonsecurity.org/PDF/NSI-White%20Paper-Web.pdf.

Mermel VL. 2004. "Old paths new directions: the use of functional foods in the treatment of obesity." *Trends Food Sci Technol* 15:532–40.

Mindell, Earl. *Dr. Earl Mindell's Amazing Apple Cider Vinegar.* New York. Contemporary Books, 2002.

Nishikawa Y, Takana Y, Nagai Y, Mori T, Kawada T, Ishihara N. 2001. "Antihypertensive effects of Kurosu extract, a traditional vinegar produced from unpolished rice, in the SHR rats." *Nippon Shokuhin Kagaku Kogaku Kaishi* 48:73–5.

Ogawa N, Satsu H, Watanabe H, Fukaya M, Tsukamoto Y, Miyamoto Y, Shimizu M. 2000b. "Acetic acid suppresses the increase in disaccharidase activity that occurs during culture of caco-2 cells." *J Nutr* 130:507–13.

Ohnami K, Matsuoka E, Okuda T. 1985. "Effects of Kurosu on the blood pressure of the spontaneously hypertension rats." *Kiso to Rinsho* 19:237–41.

Ostman E, Granfeldt Y, Persson L, Bjorck I. 2005. "Vinegar supplementation lowers glucose and insulin responses and increases satiety after a bread meal in healthy subjects." *Eur J Clin Microbiol* 59:983–8.

Rhee MS, Lee SY, Dougherty RH, Kang DH. 2003. "Antimicrobial effects of mustard flour and acetic acid against Escherichia coli O157:H7, Listeria monocytogenes, and Salmonella enterica Serovar typhimurium." *Appl Environ Microbiol* 69:2959–63.

Rutala WA, Barbee SL, Agular NC, Sobsey MD, Weber DJ. 2000. "Antimicrobial activity of home disinfectants and natural products against potential human pathogens." *Infect Control Hosp Epidemiol* 21:33–8.

Ryu JH, Deng Y, Beuchant LR. 1999. "Behavior of acid-adapted and unadapted Escherichia coli O157:H7 when exposed to reduced pH achieved with various organic acids." *J Food Prot* 62:451–5.

Sengün IY, Karabiyikli S. 2011. "Importance of acetic acid bacteria in food industry." *Food Control* 22:647–56.

Sugiyama K, Sakakibara R, Tachimoto H, Kishi M, Kaga T, Tabata I. 2009. "Effects of acetic acid bacteria supplementation on muscle damage after moderate-intensity exercise." *Anti Aging Med* 7:1–6.

Sugiyama A, Saitoh M, Takahara A, Satoh Y, Hashimoto K. 2003a. "Acute cardiovascular effects of a new beverage made of wine vinegar and grape juice, assessed using an in vivo rat." *Nutr Res* 23:1291–6.

Sugiyama M, Tang AC, Wakaki Y, Koyama W. 2003b. "Glycemic index of single and mixed meal foods among common Japanese foods with white rice as a reference food." *Eur J Clin Nutr* 57:743–52.

Trivieri, Larry Jr., editor. *Alternative Medicine: The Definitive Guide.* Berkeley, CA. Celestial Arts, 2002.

Tsuzuki W, Kikuchi Y, Shinohara K, Suzuki T. 1992. "Fluorometric assay of angiotensin I-converting enzyme inhibitory activity of vinegars." *Nippon Shokuhin Kogyo Gakkaishi* 39:188–92.

Verzelloni E, Tagliazucchi D, Conte A. 2007. "Relationship between the antioxidant properties and the phenolic and flavonoid content in traditional Balsamic vinegar." *Food Chem* 105:564–71.

Verzelloni E, Tagliazucchi D, Conte A. 2010. "From Balsamic to healthy: traditional Balsamic vinegar melanoidins inhibit lipid peroxidation during simulated gastric digestion of meat." *Food Chem Toxicol* 48:2097–102.

Yamashita H, Fujisawa K et al. 2007. "Improvement of obesity and glucose tolerance by acetate in Type 2 diabetic Otsuka Long-Evans Tokushima Fatty (OLETF) rats." *Biosci Biotechnol Biochem* 71:1236–43.

Acknowledgments

I would not have written this book but for the suggestion of my friend and publisher, Rudy Shur. Many thanks, Rudy, for your phone call to me that planted the seed and got the ball rolling. Thanks too, to your staff at Square One who were so helpful in shepherding this book all the way to its publication. Mazel tov, Amigo!

As always, my deepest thanks to, and appreciation for, my mother, brothers and sisters, nieces and nephews and their children, and all of my friends, without whom my life would be far less fun and love-filled. And to my father, for the many important lessons he taught me by his example and for the way his spirit continues to guide me since his passing from this life.

Finally, and most especially, I wish to acknowledge and thank my beloved friend and mentor Burton Goldberg for the many decades of our friendship and all I learned from him during that time. Burton passed away as I was writing this book and his sudden and unexpected passing deeply affected me, as well as so many of the countless others Burton helped guide to better health solutions over the course of his life as the "Voice of Alternative Medicine," an honorific he so rightly deserved.

It is because of Burton that I have enjoyed my long career as an author. He hired me to edit and help write the first edition of *Alternative Medicine: The Definitive Guide,* which he funded both the creation of as well as its publication. Years later, he also introduced me to Rudy, for whom I've since written many books before this one.

As I knew it would, the Guide went on to become a huge bestselling title, a feat all the more remarkable for the fact that it was self-published. Its success not only opened the door for my subsequent career, it also influenced many major traditional book publishing houses to start publishing their own books on alternative medicine and nondrug approaches to health and healing. I know this because some of my own books have been published by such houses and my editors there told me so.

Years later, Burton entrusted me to revise the Guide, which saw me expand its content by 50 percent, again as its editor, and also, this time around, its principal author. That was a task and responsibility that I relished and about which I will always have fond memories.

Burton's confidence in my abilities led him to refer to me as his "magic man." While I've always loved being called that by him, it would have been more accurate had he called me his "magician's assistant," because Burton was the one who made the real magic. Everyone who was blessed to know and love him can, along with me, attest to that fact.

Words cannot express how deeply indebted to Burton I am for all that I learned from him, and for how he recognized and brought my talents to bear in service to the joint mission we took on to help people realize that, as Burton always taught, "You don't have to be sick!" And while a book on apple cider vinegar hardly matches the scope and depth of the books I created with Burton and on my own and as a co-author with others, its subject matter is exactly the type of thing Burton would have appreciated because of the many health benefits ACV can provide.

Thank you, Burton, with love, always!

About the Author

Larry Trivieri Jr is a bestselling author and nationally recognized lay authority on holistic, integrative, and non-drug-based healing methods, with more than 30 years of personal experience in exploring techniques for optimal wellness and human transformation, including acid-alkaline balance. During that time, Trivieri has interviewed and studied with over 400 of the world's top physicians and other health practitioners in over 50 disciplines in the holistic health field.

Trivieri is the author or co-author of more than 20 books on health, including *The Acid-Alkaline Lifestyle, The Acid-Alkaline Food Guide, Juice Alive, The American Holistic Medical Association Guide to Holistic Health, The Self-Care Guide to Holistic Medicine,* and *Health On The Edge: Visionary Views of Healing in the New Millennium.* He also served as editor and principal writer of both editions of the landmark health encyclopedia, *Alternative Medicine: The Definitive Guide,* and has written over 200 articles for Internet-based health sites, including 1HealthyWorld.com and IntegrativeHealthReview.com. He has also written numerous feature articles for a variety of publications, including *Alternative Medicine,* for which he also served as contributing editor from 1999 through 2002; *Natural Health, Natural Solutions,* and *Yoga Journal.* He has also been written about in a number of national publications, including *The Washington Post.*

Trivieri is dedicated to sharing the wealth of potentially life-saving information he has learned about with as wide an audience as possible in order to help usher in a new era of wellness and health care in the 21st century. To that end, he also lectures about health nationwide, and has been a featured guest on numerous TV and radio shows across the United States.

Trivieri is also an acclaimed novelist and the author of *The Monster and Freddie Fype,* as well as the forthcoming titles *Krystle's Quest and Tommy's Big Question.* While continuing to write about health-related topics, he is also at work on another novel and resides in upstate New York.

Index

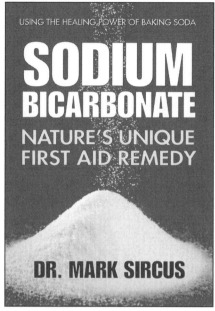

SODIUM BICARBONATE

Nature's Unique First Aid Remedy

Dr. Mark Sircus

What if there were a natural health-promoting substance that was inexpensive, available at any grocery store in the country, and probably sitting in your cupboard right now? There is.

It is called sodium bicarbonate, although you may know it as baking soda. For years, sodium bicarbonate has been used on a daily basis as part of a number of hospital treatments, but most people remain unaware of its full therapeutic potential. In his new book, Dr. Mark Sircus shows how this common compound may be used in the alleviation, or possibly even prevention, of many forms of illness.

Sodium Bicarbonate begins with a basic overview of the everyday item known as baking soda, chronicling its long history of use as an effective home remedy. It then explains the role sodium bicarbonate plays in achieving optimal pH balance, which is revealed as an important factor in maintaining good health. The book goes on to detail how sodium bicarbonate and its effect on pH may benefit sufferers of a number of conditions, including kidney disease, fungal infection, influenza, hypertension, and even cancer. Finally, it lists the various ways in which sodium bicarbonate may be taken, suggesting the easiest and most effective method for your situation.

By providing a modern approach to this time-honored remedy, *Sodium Bicarbonate* illustrates the need to see baking soda in a whole new light. While it was once considered simply an ingredient in baked goods and toothpaste, sodium bicarbonate contains powerful properties that may help you balance your system, regain your well-being, and avoid future health problems.

$16.95 • 208 pages • 6 x 9-inch paperback • ISBN 978-0-7570-0394-3

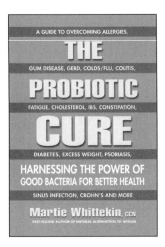

THE PROBIOTIC CURE

Harnessing the Power of Good Bacteria for Better Health

Martie Whittekin, CCN

Only recently have scientists recognized that an imbalance in the bacteria of your stomach can cause a host of serious disorders, from diabetes to ulcers. Now, best-selling health author Martie Whittekin has written *The Probiotic Cure,* a guide to overcoming many of our most common health issues.

Part One of *The Probiotic Cure* explains how our internal flora works to promote health and how it can become unbalanced due to a poor diet, medications, and other factors. It goes on to explain how this balance can be restored safely and effectively by using probiotics—good bacteria available in supplement form. Part Two discusses the most common health disorders that may arise from a bacterial imbalance and explains both conventional treatments and the probiotics approach to healing.

$16.95 • 176 pages • 6 x 9-inch paperback • ISBN 978-0-7570-0423-0

THE MAGNESIUM SOLUTION FOR HIGH BLOOD PRESSURE

How to Use Magnesium to Help Prevent & Relieve Hypertension Naturally

Jay S. Cohen, MD

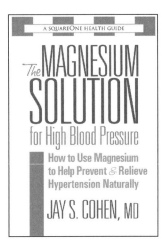

Approximately 50 percent of Americans have hypertension. Many medications are available to combat this condition, but they come with potential side effects. Fortunately, there is a remedy that's both safe and effective—magnesium. *The Magnesium Solution for High Blood Pressure* describes the best types of magnesium, explores appropriate dosage, and details the use of magnesium with hypertension meds.

$5.95 • 96 pages • 4 x 7-inch mass paperback • ISBN 978-0-7570-0255-7

ANTI-INFLAMMATORY OXYGEN THERAPY

Your Complete Guide to Understanding and Using Natural Oxygen Therapy

Dr. Mark Sircus

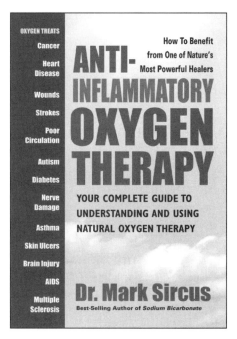

It is invisible, it is powerful, and it is life sustaining. It is oxygen. We inhale it every day of our lives, and while it makes up only 21 percent of the air we breathe, it is the key to our very existence. The more we learn about its healing properties, the more we recognize its tremendous potential as a medical treatment for many serious disorders. Yet few have known about its important therapeutic uses—until now. In *Anti-Inflammatory Oxygen Therapy,* best-selling author Dr. Mark Sircus examines the remarkable benefits oxygen therapy offers, from detoxification to treatments for a wide variety of disorders—from aging to gastric disorders to cancer.

While the term "oxygen therapy" conjures images of crucially ill patients lying in hospital beds with tubes strapped to their faces, this book will show that oxygen can offer so much more. Dr. Sircus first looks at the nature of oxygen and its purpose in the body. He then provides an understanding of how inflammation works to destroy the body's tissues over time, and how oxygen can reverse this process. He examines the current treatments that use hyperbaric oxygen chambers as well as newer protocols that employ this vital element. In addition, Dr. Sircus offers a simple, safe, and highly effective fifteen-minute technique that can be used in the privacy of your home so that you can enjoy maximum benefits for a healthier life.

If you are wondering why you haven't heard about this "miracle" treatment before, the fact is oxygen cannot be patented, it is not expensive, and you don't have to be a specialist to use it. Without a tremendous profit behind it, it's become a well-kept secret, but the facts speak for themselves. In this book, you will learn these life-altering facts—information that could change your health for the better.

$15.95 • 192 pages • 6 x 9-inch paperback • ISBN 978-0-7570-0415-5

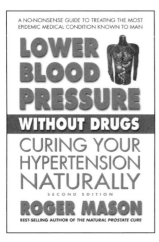

LOWER BLOOD PRESSURE WITHOUT DRUGS

SECOND EDITION

Curing Your Hypertension Naturally

Roger Mason

Over 65 million Americans have high blood pressure. Although prescription drugs may effectively treat this disorder, they can have dangerous side effects. Fortunately, natural alternatives are available.

In this updated edition of *Lower Blood Pressure Without Drugs,* best-selling author Roger Mason offers a nutritional approach to managing hypertension safely and naturally. First, you'll learn all about high blood pressure—what it is, what causes it, and how it is diagnosed. Then, you'll discover how a simple diet, rich in whole grains and low in fat, can improve both blood pressure and general health.

$9.95 • 128 pages • 6 x 9-inch paperback • ISBN 978-0-7570-0366-0

LOWER YOUR CHOLESTEROL WITHOUT DRUGS

SECOND EDITION

Curing High Cholesterol Naturally

Roger Mason

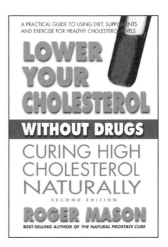

According to the American Heart Association, high cholesterol is the leading cause of coronary heart disease. While prescription drugs can lower cholesterol, they can also have undesired effects. But is a better option available?

In *Lower Your Cholesterol Without Drugs,* Roger Mason offers you a safe, effective way to treat this condition and improve your health. The book looks at the causes of high cholesterol and then explains how a balanced, vitamin-rich diet can lower cholesterol while enhancing your well-being. Information is also provided on natural supplements that can help lower even genetically high cholesterol.

$9.95 • 128 pages • 6 x 9-inch paperback • ISBN 978-0-7570-0367-7

YOUR BLOOD NEVER LIES

How to Read a Blood Test for a Longer, Healthier Life

James B. LaValle, RPh, CCN

If you're like most people, you probably rely on your doctor to interpret the results of your blood tests, which contain a wealth of information on the state of your health. A blood test can tell you how well your liver and kidneys are functioning, your potential for heart disease and diabetes, the strength of your immune system, the chemical profile of your blood, and many other important facts about the state of your health. And yet, most of us cannot decipher these results ourselves, nor can we even formulate the right questions to ask about them— or we couldn't, until now.

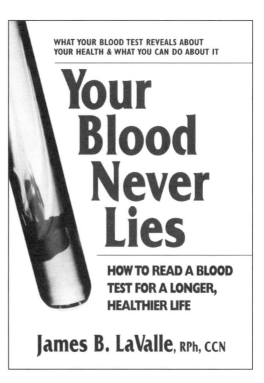

WHAT YOUR BLOOD TEST REVEALS ABOUT YOUR HEALTH & WHAT YOU CAN DO ABOUT IT

Your Blood Never Lies

HOW TO READ A BLOOD TEST FOR A LONGER, HEALTHIER LIFE

James B. LaValle, RPh, CCN

In *Your Blood Never Lies,* best-selling author Dr. James LaValle clears the mystery surrounding blood test results. In simple language, he explains all the information found on a typical lab report—the medical terminology, the numbers and percentages, and the laboratory jargon—and makes it accessible. This means that you will be able to look at your own blood test results and understand the significance of each biological marker being measured. To help you take charge of your health, Dr. LaValle also recommends the most effective standard and complementary treatments for dealing with any problematic findings. Rounding out the book are explanations of lab values that do not appear on the standard blood test, but that should be requested for a more complete picture of your current physiological condition.

A blood test can reveal so much about your body, but only if you can interpret the results. *Your Blood Never Lies* provides the up-to-date information you need to understand your results and take control of your life.

$16.95 • 368 pages • 6 x 9-inch paperback • ISBN 978-0-7570-0350-9

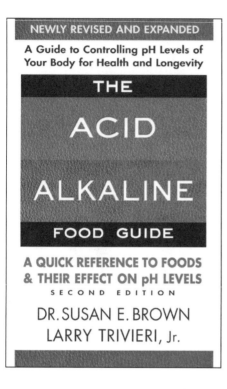

NEWLY REVISED AND EXPANDED

A Guide to Controlling pH Levels of Your Body for Health and Longevity

THE

ACID

ALKALINE

FOOD GUIDE

A QUICK REFERENCE TO FOODS & THEIR EFFECT ON pH LEVELS

SECOND EDITION

DR. SUSAN E. BROWN

LARRY TRIVIERI, Jr.

THE ACID-ALKALINE FOOD GUIDE,
SECOND EDITION

A Quick Reference to Foods & Their Effect on pH Levels

Susan Brown, PhD, and Larry Trivieri, Jr.

In the last few years, researchers around the world have increasingly reported the importance of acid-alkaline balance. *The Acid-Alkaline Food Guide* was designed as an easy-to-follow guide to the most common foods that influence your body's pH level. Now in its Second Edition, this bestseller has been expanded to include many more domestic and international foods. Updated information also explores (and refutes) the myths about pH balance and diet, and guides the reader to supplements that can help the body achieve a healthy pH level.

The Acid-Alkaline Food Guide begins by explaining how the acid-alkaline environment of the body is influenced by foods. It then presents a list of thousands of foods and their acid-alkaline effects. Included are not only single foods, such as fruits and vegetables, but also popular combination and even common fast foods. In each case, you'll not only discover whether a food is acidifying or alkalizing, but also learn the degree to which that food affects the body. Informative insets guide you in choosing the food that's right for you.

The first book of its kind—now updated and expanded—*The Acid-Alkaline Food Guide* will quickly become the resource you turn to at home, in restaurants, and whenever you want to select a food that can help you reach your health and dietary goals.

8.95 • 224 pages • 4 x 7-inch paperback • ISBN 978-0-7570-0393-6

Unsafe at Any Meal

What the FDA Does Not Want You to Know About the Foods You Eat

Dr. Renee Joy Dufault

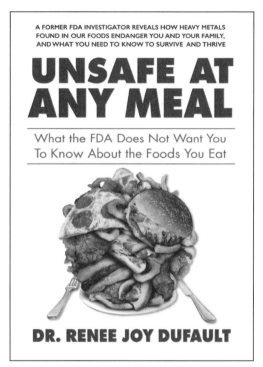

A FORMER FDA INVESTIGATOR REVEALS HOW HEAVY METALS FOUND IN OUR FOODS ENDANGER YOU AND YOUR FAMILY, AND WHAT YOU NEED TO KNOW TO SURVIVE AND THRIVE

UNSAFE AT ANY MEAL

What the FDA Does Not Want You To Know About the Foods You Eat

DR. RENEE JOY DUFAULT

Each year, Americans consume food products that contain heavy metals, pesticides, and harmful additives—with the blessing of the FDA. Why is this happening and why haven't you heard about it? In *Unsafe at Any Meal,* Dr. Renee Dufault, former food investigator for the Food and Drug Administration, provides the startling answers. While at the FDA, Dr. Dufault discovered toxic mercury residue in the plumbing systems of food manufacturing plants and in processed foods sold in supermarkets. When Dr. Dufault revealed these disturbing findings to her superiors, she was told to stop her investigation. She retired early and devoted her energy to making the public aware of the insidious dangers that contaminate our food. To expose what still seems to be a well-kept secret by the FDA, she has written *Unsafe at Any Meal* to provide consumers with the information they need to know.

Over fifty years ago, Rachel Carson's book *Silent Spring* exposed the dangers of DDT in our food supply. Unfortunately, it seems that the problem of food contamination has actually become worse. Backed by research and first-hand experience, Dr. Dufault reveals how the FDA has failed us, and outlines how you can protect yourself and your family by filling your kitchen with food that is free of toxic substances.

$16.95 • 192 pages • 6 x 9-inch paperback • ISBN 978-0-7570-0436-0

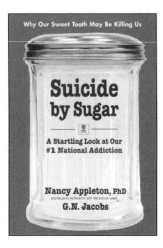

SUICIDE BY SUGAR

A Startling Look at Our #1 National Addiction

Nancy Appleton, PhD, and G.N. Jacobs

More than two decades ago, Nancy Appleton's *Lick the Sugar Habit* exposed the health dangers of America's high-sugar diet. Now, in *Suicide by Sugar,* Appleton, along with journalist G.N. Jacobs, presents a broader view of the problems caused by our favorite ingredient.

The authors offer startling facts that link a range of disorders—from dementia and hypoglycemia to obesity and cancer—to our growing addiction to sugar. Rounding out the book is a sound diet plan along with a number of recipes for sweet, easy-to-prepare delectable dishes, all made without sugar or fruit.

$15.95 • 192 pages • 6 x 9-inch paperback • ISBN 978-0-7570-0306-6

HEALTH AT GUNPOINT

The FDA's Silent War Against Health Freedom

James J. Gormley

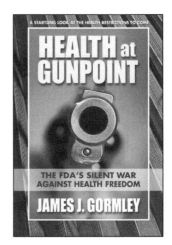

While the original intent of the Food and Drug Administration may have been honorable, over time, unfortunately, the mission has become tainted by lobbyists. *Health at Gunpoint* presents a history of the agency's long battle against health products and examines some of its most controversial decisions.

Now, the FDA is again poised to make decisions that would have a major impact on the public, this time, by imposing restrictions that could eliminate many of the nutritional supplements we take. *Health at Gunpoint* not only sheds light on what is happening, but also prepares us for the coming battle.

$14.95 • 176 pages • 6 x 9-inch paperback • ISBN 978-0-7570-0381-3

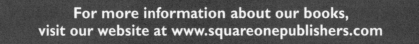